Managing Family Planning in General Practice

Sam Rowlands
General Practitioner
Bedfordshire

With contributions by

Shelley Mehigan

Catriona Sutherland

and

Maggie Pettifer

Foreword by

Yvonne Carter
Professor of General Practice and Primary Care
St Bartholomew's and The Royal London School
of Medicine and Dentistry

Radcliffe Medical Press

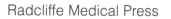

Radcliffe Medical Press Ltd
18 Marcham Road, Abingdon, Oxon OX14 1AA, UK

Radcliffe Medical Press, Inc.
141 Fifth Avenue, New York, NY 10010, USA

British Library Cataloguing in Publication Data

A catalogue record for this book is available from the British Library.

ISBN 1 85775 205 8

Library of Congress Cataloging-in-Publication Data is available.

Typeset by Advance Typesetting Ltd, Oxfordshire
Printed and bound by Biddles Ltd, Guildford and King's Lynn

About the author

Sam Rowlands, MRCGP, MFFP, DCH, DRCOG, has been a full-time principal in general practice in Biggleswade, Bedfordshire for 15 years, a GP trainer for the past 12 years and a GP vocational training scheme course organizer for four years.

He was born in the London Hospital (as it was then) – which makes him a Cockney – and like his father before him, he studied medicine at the London Hospital. He became interested in family planning while a clinical student and was much inspired by Dr Katie Schöpflin, who was a GP family planner, practising in the East End of London at the time. After completing a training scheme for general practice based in Redhill, Surrey, he was research assistant at the Margaret Pyke Centre, London, where he conducted studies on emergency contraception.

Sam Rowlands was approved as a family planning instructing doctor in GP premises 12 years ago and has been a principal investigator for the UK Family Planning Research Network, University of Exeter, for the last eight years. He is currently chairman of the Faculty of Family Planning and Reproductive Health Care of the RCOG, and sits on the Medical Advisory Committees of both the Family Planning Association and Brook Advisory Centres.

Contents

List of contributors   xi

Acknowledgements   xiii

Foreword   xv

Preface   xvii

List of abbreviations   xix

1   Family planning in the UK – a public health perspective   1
    Figures for a model practice   1
    Needs assessment   2
    Commissioning services   3
    An ideal family planning service   4
    Cost–benefit analysis   5
    Targets   5
    Outcome indicators   6

2   Trends in family planning in the UK   9
    The GP family planning service   9
    Preferred source of outlet   9
    Contraceptive usage in the UK   10
    The media   11
    Pill scares   12
    Abortion – trends   15
    Summary   16

3   How to set up a family planning service in general practice   17
    Regulations   17

Guidelines   17
Women's choice of service   18
Young people   18
A dedicated clinic?   20
Premises and equipment   21
Choice of method offered   22
Monitoring of patients   23
Method teaching   23
Claim forms and fees   26
Abortion   28
Recall   28
Publicity   29
Expanding and improving the service   30
Financial aspects   30

4   The role of the practice nurse
    Shelley Mehigan and Catriona Sutherland   33
        The development of practice nursing   33
        Underused and undervalued   34
        Accessibility   35
        Young people   35
        Education   36
        Role development   38
        Pill checks   39
        Nurse reissuing of contraceptives   39
        Telephone advice   40
        Emergency contraception   41
        Counselling   41
        Female barrier methods   42
        The practice nurse as a resource   42
        Teamwork   43
        Confidentiality   43
        Legal issues and accountability   44

5   The role of other key members of the
    primary health care team   45
        Practice manager   45

Health visitor 45
Midwife 46
School nurse 46
Receptionist 47

6 Family planning outside the practice setting 49
Family planning clinics 49
Gynaecologists 49
Accident and emergency departments 50
Genitourinary medicine 50
Young persons' centres 50
Schools 51
Health promotion unit 51
Health authority 51
Charitable organizations 51
Brook Advisory Centres 52
Pharmacists 52

7 Information technology 55
Faxes 55
Trends in general practice computing 55
The consultation 57
Prescribing 57
Practice administration 58
Training 58
Electronic data interchange 58

8 Planning for patient-centred care
Maggie Pettifer 61
Where are we now? 62
Planning the future of the service 68
Promoting your improved family planning service 70
Planning pays off 71

9 Quality issues 73
Clinical effectiveness 73
Protocols (local guidelines) 74

Evidence-based medicine	74
Audit	77
Setting standards	80
Training of general practitioners	80
Training of other members of the PHCT	81
Teaching	82
Research	82

10 Methods of contraception – administrative aspects — 85

Personally administered items	85
The Drug Tariff	86
Pills	86
Injectables	87
Subdermal implants	87
Intrauterine devices	88
The intrauterine system (IUS)	89
Caps and diaphragms	89
Spermicides	90
Condoms	90
Methods only available in family planning clinics	91
Methods available from the pharmacist	91
Emergency contraception	91
Vasectomy	92
Female sterilization	92

11 Counselling for unwanted pregnancy and sterilization — 93

Counselling for unwanted pregnancy	93
Counselling for sterilization	94

12 Medico-legal and ethical issues — 97

Human rights	97
Confidentiality	98
Consent	99
Sterilization of those with learning difficulties	101
Vasectomy	101

IUDs 101
The combined pill 102
Abortion 102
Negligence 103
Intimate examinations 104
Access to medical records 105

13 The future 107
A nurse-led service 107
Generalists or specialists? 107
Training issues 108
Accessibility 108
The role of the pharmacist 109
Convergence of services 109
Funding 109
The Department for Education and Employment 110
The implications of new technologies 110
The team approach 110
Attitudes 111

References and further reading 113
References 113
Further reading 118

Useful addresses 119

Appendix 1 Example of a patient questionnaire 121

Appendix 2 Protocol for the administration of
injectable contraceptives 125

Index 129

List of contributors

Shelley Mehigan is a clinical nurse specialist in family planning. She works at the first fully-integrated sexual health service in this country in East Berkshire and runs a family planning clinic in general practice in Maidenhead.

After qualifying in general and occupational health nursing, Shelley started work as a practice nurse in 1980. Since specializing in family planning she has worked in both areas and has been involved for a number of years with family planning training in Berkshire. She is also nurse advisor to the Breast Care Campaign.

Shelley is currently the chair of the Family Planning Forum at the Royal College of Nursing.

Catriona Sutherland is a registered nurse and has worked for a number of years in family planning, having undertaken advanced training in family planning and women's health. She has worked in a variety of settings including hospital and community clinics, in specialist youth advisory clinics, as an abortion counsellor and as a domiciliary family planning nurse. Since 1989 she has been a practice nurse, qualified to work as a nurse specialist in family planning and women's health. She is a member of the RCN Family Planning Forum steering group.

Maggie Pettifer is a healthcare communication consultant and writer.

Acknowledgements

Numerous individuals and organizations have helped me assemble the ideas and information in this book. I would specifically like to thank Toni Belfield (Director of Information at the Family Planning Association) and Jane Urwin (Information Officer at the FPA) for their helpful comments. Dr Stephen Gillam, Consultant in Public Health Medicine at Bedfordshire Health, helped with Chapters 1 and 9. Shelley Mehigan and Catriona Sutherland, as well as writing Chapter 4 so well, made sure I considered the nurse's point of view throughout. Maggie Pettifer contributed Chapter 8 which has certainly added a new dimension to family planning for me; she also made my English a lot plainer and helped with the overall plan of the book, finally knocking the manuscript into shape before submission.

Foreword

The importance of family planning in general practice has been emphasized in recent years. This book is designed for general practitioners and members of primary health care teams who wish to embark on improving their knowledge and skills in this area. It will particularly help GPs and practice nurses respond to the challenge of keeping up-to-date. All practices should examine this aspect of their work to ensure that their patients have access to a high quality family planning service. It is important that we enable our patients to make informed decisions in relation to family planning. This book is both timely and necessary.

It is always encouraging when a professional with a long-term interest in a subject wants to share his/her enthusiasm. It is especially so when the result is a publication such as this. Sam Rowlands has a background in general practice, postgraduate education and family planning. Clearly committed to quality and high standards of patient care, he has described an approach to managing family planning in general practice using practical aspects in a clear and easy to follow way, making use of references, diagrams and bullet points where appropriate. Good history taking, sensitive examination techniques, negotiated management plans, well kept clinical records and equitable access to services are integral parts of our work in this area. Emphasis is given to patient-centred care, teamwork and training.

The author and other contributors are particularly well placed to guide the reader. Perhaps, more importantly, they are experienced in day-to-day clinical care. They have gathered together an impressive array of topics ranging from basic practice administration and finance to new developments in information technology and commissioning of care. Whilst the benefits of evidence-based health care and clinical effectiveness are acknowledged, gaps in general practice-based research are highlighted. The evolving role of the practice nurse is also emphasized.

This book is easy to understand and guides the reader through the range of skills necessary for an understanding of family planning, the management of specific conditions, the ethical dilemmas and the medico-legal pitfalls in relation to this area.

There is much that can be achieved in general practice in this area. This book addresses some of the most pertinent issues. I congratulate the author on his far-sightedness and expertise in producing it.

Yvonne Carter
March 1997

Preface

There are many books about family planning. Most of them tell readers about the different contraceptive methods in more or less detail. Those professing to be about family planning in general practice (not all of them written by authors who are general practitioners) do not tell you how to *provide* the service. To fill this gap I have therefore written a very practical book about *how* to manage a family planning service in general practice. Intentionally it includes very little on the technical and scientific aspects of the contraceptives themselves.

It is difficult to define the scope of family planning. The book does not set out to encompass *all* of reproductive health care. The menopause has now become a big topic in its own right. Similarly, infertility is a very broad topic outside the scope of this text. Screening of breasts and cervix may often take place within family planning consultations, but there are good texts already written on this. Sexual health includes sexuality and sexually transmitted infections – a companion book in this series, *Sexual health promotion in general practice*, is already published.

This book concentrates on the unique features of family planning when practised in a general practice context, and how to manage a service for those men and women of reproductive age registered with the practice – and possibly for those not registered too. I have tried to be as up to date as possible to help the primary health care team cope with the practice in the ever changing NHS, and have included chapters on quality, information technology and healthy alliances with those relevant specialists and agencies outside the practice. There is also a chapter on the population-based public health approach to family planning which is ever more necessary in an era of involvement in commissioning of services.

This book will, I hope, be invaluable for practice nurses and GPs, and also for other members of the primary health care team involved in running family planning services. It will be particularly helpful for those launching a new service and those re-evaluating an existing service.

Sam Rowlands
March 1997

List of abbreviations

A&E	Accident and Emergency
BMA	British Medical Association
CD-ROM	Compact disk read-only memory
CES	Contraceptive Education Service
CSM	Committee on Safety of Medicines
DOH	Department of Health
ENB	English National Board
FP10	(Prescription form used by GPs)
FPA	Family Planning Association
GMC	General Medical Council
GMSC	General Medical Services Committee
GP	General practitioner
HA	Health authority (fusion of former district health authorities and family health services authorities)
HEA	Health Education Authority
HIV	Human immunodeficiency virus
IUD	Intrauterine device
IUS	Intrauterine system
JCC	Joint Committee on Contraception
JCPTGP	Joint Committee for Postgraduate Training in General Practice
LMC	Local Medical Committee
NHS	National Health Service
OTC	Over the counter
P	Pharmacy
PACT	Prescribing analyses and cost tabulations
PC	Personal computer
PHCT	Primary health care team
POM	Prescription only medicine
RCN	Royal College of Nursing
R&D	Research and development
RCGP	Royal College of General Practitioners
RCOG	Royal College of Obstetricians and Gynaecologists
SHO	Senior House Officer

STI	Sexually transmitted infection
TOP	Termination of pregnancy
UKCC	United Kingdom Central Council
VAT	Value added tax

Family planning in the UK – a public health perspective

The objective of family planning from a population perspective is to support sexually active individuals in enjoying the positive aspects of their sexuality without detriment to their health and to enable women to have the number of children that they desire when they wish to have them.[1] An implicit aim of public policy in England and Wales is that each pregnancy should be both planned and wanted. We are clearly a long way from this situation, and family planning services in general practice have a large part to play in trying to achieve this aim. As will be mentioned in Chapter 2, one in three births are unplanned, and one in five of all pregnancies end in induced abortion.

Figures for a model practice

According to 1996 British Medical Association (BMA) data, the average list size of a GP is about 1900 patients. The mean number of GPs per practice is 2.75. A group practice caring for a population of 10 000 patients will be taken as the demographic unit for primary health care. An average practice will comprise 51% females and 49% males.

Of the 5100 females in the practice, 2430 will be women aged 15–49. Using figures from the 1993 *General household survey*. The current fertility status of this age group can be estimated as follows:[2]

- using reversible contraception   1148

- sterilized, or partner sterilized   568

- sterile after another operation   48

- pregnant/trying to conceive   194

- no partner   360

- menopause/possibly infertile   108

- just does not like contraception   4

Total   2430.

Of the 1148 women using reversible contraception, about 453 will be using non-medical methods and the other 695 will be under medical supervision.

National statistics for the prevalence of consultations on contraceptive management[3] indicate the following:

- females aged 16–24 consulting per 10 000
  per year   = 4707

- number of female consultations in age group
  16–24 with a doctor per 10 000 per year   = 7637

therefore

- average number of consultations per female
  patient aged 16–24 per year   =   1.5.

Incidence data for this population of 10 000 for a period of 1 year would be:

- live births   131

- therapeutic abortions   30.

Currently 89% of abortions carried out on women resident in England and Wales are undertaken at less than 13 weeks' gestation (39% at less than 9 weeks). Sixty-seven per cent of abortions are paid for by the NHS in England and Wales (this includes some abortions carried out in the private sector under agency arrangements) although there is wide variation between health authorities. In Scotland, 95% of abortions are provided by the NHS.

Needs assessment

The above figures, based on national data, give some idea of the family planning needs of the women in a general practice. By referring to the annual reports of the Director of Public Health of the health authority these figures can be scaled down for one's own practice locality. Furthermore, using a practice information system with accurate coding, a breakdown can be built up which is practice-specific. For example, a practice that has 25% of its list comprising females aged 15–44 will need a higher level of family planning activity than a practice with 15%.

The preferences of local people should be taken into account. These preferences will very much depend on local factors in the area of the practice: ethnic groups, socio-economic factors and geography of the practice area.

Methods made available and style of provision should be tailored to the needs of one's own practice population and that of the locality. For example, the needs of inner-city Liverpool are very different from the needs in the Scottish Highlands. Needs assessment should allow the primary health care team (PHCT) to look at both its own service provision and the commissioning from other providers. It also allows GPs to be involved in the allocation of resources, irrespective of whether they are fundholders or not. Many non-fundholders have their say through dialogue with commissioners at locality planning meetings.

It can be useful for GPs to work with trust providers in assessing needs in their locality. There should be collaboration between the PHCT, other family planning service providers and commissioners on needs assessment and commissioning. The potential conflict of interest for GPs who are in a position both of providing a service and purchasing it from others must be recognized.

Commissioning services

General practices can be involved in commissioning in different ways. A unified commissioning project in Barking and Havering identified deficiencies in existing family planning services. A service specification was drawn up which included the range of services to be offered, targets to be achieved in 1 year and 5 years, quality standards and monitoring arrangements. Tenders were invited which had to include operational protocols, a named person responsible for the delivery, accessibility and quality of the service and quality markers. A general practice won a contract for one locality and provides the service to the population of this geographical area.

Since fundholding began in 1991, fundholders have been responsible for commissioning vasectomy and female sterilization. Provision
of vasectomy appears to have improved considerably since the situation in the late 1980s when many district health authorities had
almost ceased to make provision, and a few NHS vasectomies were
performed in hospital operating theatres and family planning clinics.
An Executive Letter was sent to all managers in 1991 reminding them
of their obligation to provide sterilizations on grounds other than
purely medical ones, and the purchaser–provider arrangements seem
to have coped with this in most areas. Some purchasers however
have of late been looking at vasectomy, along with other procedures,
as targets for complete withdrawal of funding. Vasectomy arrangements are discussed further in Chapter 10.

Since April 1996, fundholders have had the responsibility for purchasing abortion services, unless it is decided for reasons of con-
science on the part of all partners that they want to opt out.[4] Further
information on the medico-legal and ethical issues raised by abortion
is given in Chapter 12. The abortion provider will often be the local
gynaecology department of the acute trust or family planning department of the community trust. Second-trimester abortions may be
better referred to a charitable organization.

With the advent of total purchasing in 1994 (still only a pilot project) there have been concerns about whether GPs will purchase part
of the service from trust family planning clinics. In West Berkshire,
for example, some clinics have been threatened with 'rationalization'. Total purchasing tends to encourage collaboration between
practices so that it becomes, in effect, locality commissioning. How
this develops remains to be seen. All one can say at present is that
these GPs operate under the same rules as health authorities and if
national regulations and guidance are not adhered to then their
continuance in the scheme may be stopped by regions.

An ideal family planning service

If uptake of contraceptive services in a practice is to reach the maximum level possible the following criteria must be met. The contraceptive service (information, advice and clinical component) must:

• be accessible at times most convenient to users and potential
  users

- provide a full range of methods

- offer a choice of appointment and drop-in systems

- offer patients the choice to consult female GPs and practice nurses

- be (and be perceived to be) private and confidential

- offer anonymity where this is required

- be designed, delivered and developed on the basis of local needs assessment (which includes the views of non-users as well as of service users)

- address the diversity of sexual and reproductive health care need within the community

- be widely and effectively advertised.

These criteria, adapted from Walsh *et al.* (1996),[5] should be reviewed as part of the business planning process described in Chapter 8. The overall ethos of a family planning service must incorporate certain basic human rights (see Chapter 8).

Cost–benefit analysis

Family planning services are inexpensive in terms of total NHS expenditure, comprising only 0.5% of total public expenditure on health care in Great Britain in 1991.[6] The existing use of NHS family planning services results in the avoidance of over 3 million unplanned pregnancies in Great Britain each year, representing a direct saving of £2.6 billion per annum. Adding indirect social security costs, this saving becomes £25 billion per annum. This gives an overall financial benefit-to-cost ratio of 11:1; that is, for every £100 spent on family planning services the public sector can expect a benefit of £1100.

Targets

The *Health of the Nation* target is an indicator of success or other- wise in the general objective of reducing the number of unintended pregnancies. The target is to reduce the rate of conception in the under-16s in England by at least 50% by the year 2000 (from 9.5 per

1000 girls aged 13–15 in 1989 to no more than 4.8 per 1000). The figure had come down to 8.1 per 1000 in 1993 but rose slightly to 8.3 per 1000 in 1994. District health authority under-16 conception rates are also available for the period 1992–4, which will be helpful to look at. Similar reports to the *Health of the Nation* – setting out health strategies, objectives and targets with a section on sexual health – were published in Wales and Northern Ireland.

The pregnancy rate of 16 to 19-year-olds is also important and is a useful and sensitive indicator of the effectiveness of health education and youth advisory and contraceptive services, and much greater numbers are involved.

Outcome indicators

To ensure that the services provided are as effective as possible and that our patients obtain optimal results, four performance indicators measuring the outcome of family planning services have been developed.[7] All four indicators assume uniform access to abortion. A worked example is given for the first two indicators (Tables 1.1 and 1.2), based on a practice with 10 000 patients.

1 Total period legal abortion rate.
This rate represents the average number of abortions that would occur per woman in the practice, if women experienced the practice's

Table 1.1: Worked example

Age group	No. TOPs*	No. females	Rate per 1000	No. years each woman in age group	No. TOPs per 1000 women during years in age group
15–19	5	281	17.8	5	89.0
20–24	9	342	26.3	5	131.5
25–29	7	396	17.7	5	88.5
30–34	5	392	12.8	5	64.0
35–39	3	342	8.8	5	44.0
40–44	1	327	3.1	5	15.5
Total	30	2080		30	432.5

*Taken from 3-year moving average, using figures from current year and previous two years. Total period abortion rate per woman is 0.43, i.e. on average, likelihood of any woman having a termination of pregnancy (TOP) during her reproductive life is 43%.

age-specific abortion rates of the calendar year in question throughout their childbearing age span of 15 to 44 years.

2 Total period legal abortion rate as a percentage of the crude potential fertility rate.

The crude potential fertility rate is the total period legal abortion rate added to the total period fertility rate. The total period fertility rate is the average number of live births that would occur per woman in the practice if women experienced the practice's current age-specific fertility rates throughout their childbearing age. Miscarriages and stillbirths are not included in the crude potential fertility rate.

Table 1.2: Worked example

Age group	No. live births	No. females	Rate per 1000	No. years each woman in age group	No. live births per 1000 women during years in age group
15–19	9	281	32.0	5	160.0
20–24	30	342	87.7	5	438.5
25–29	46	396	116.2	5	581.0
30–34	33	392	84.2	5	421.0
35–39	11	342	32.2	5	161.0
40–44	2	327	6.1	5	30.5
Total	131	2080		30	1792.0

Total period fertility rate per woman = 1.79, i.e. on average, number of live births any woman is likely to have during her reproductive life = 1.79.
Crude potential fertility rate = 0.43 + 1.79 = 2.22.
$\frac{0.43}{2.22} \times 100 = 19\%$

3 The proportion of terminations performed after 12 weeks' gestation.

4 Conception rates for those aged under 16.

This performance indicator needs to include a proportion of the live births and abortions occurring in 16-year-olds, as these girls conceived when they were still aged 15. This is important to remember if practice data are to be compared with the national average.

As a rougher outcome guide – which includes less bother in calculation – in a practice where the number of patients and the age distribution are relatively stable, the number of terminations can be used to look at changes over time in that practice. In that case, it would be best to take a 3-year moving average to iron out the effect of small numbers.

Disadvantages of using data from a single practice

There is some doubt about the statistical validity of using data at practice level as the denominator is small. Aggregating data from several practices is better. The statistical validity may also be improved by aggregating data from one practice over several years. The public health medicine specialist responsible for community services will be able to advise on matters such as this.

Are these performance indicators sufficient?

To use only the above performance indicators would be dangerous. Much of the work carried out in contraceptive consultations involves counselling about sexuality, psychosexual difficulties and other emotional aspects of reproduction. Assessing performance in these areas by qualitative techniques is problematic. Nevertheless, some attempt should be made to do this; quantitative measures do not reflect the service in its entirety.

2

Trends in family planning in the UK

The GP family planning service

It seems strange now to think that intrauterine devices (IUDs) and diaphragms could not be prescribed on an FP10 before 1973. Since GPs entered the free NHS family planning services on 1 July 1975, they have become a major source of contraceptive advice in the UK.[8]

Over these two decades, provision of contraceptive care has shifted from clinics to general practice; the ratio of general practice to clinic attendances has increased from 0.9:1 to 2.3:1. It is difficult to say how much this trend is due to changing consumer preference, family planning clinic closures and cut-backs or to GPs improving and promoting their services. During this time employment of practice nurses has become the norm, and many group practices have a GP and/or nurse who specialize in family planning, offering female barrier methods and IUD insertion. Some practices now offer vasectomy too.

Preferred source of outlet

A survey in my practice in Bedfordshire of all women aged 20–49[9] showed current sources of contraceptive supplies were:

- own GP   59%
- over-the-counter   26%
- family planning clinic   11%
- mail order   2%
- other   2%.

It is important to realize that, based on this survey in my practice, about 30% of women choose methods which are not medically dependent, but within this 30%, some women may seek the advice of their pharmacist. Forty-one per cent of women go outside the practice for advice.

If the aim of your practice is to encourage patients who seek advice outside to consult within the practice, the reasons why they go elsewhere will need to be examined. However, an individual must never be pressurized into accepting contraceptive care from an outlet they are not comfortable with. This is discussed further in Chapter 3. Use of surveys and questionnaires is discussed in Chapter 8.

Contraceptive usage in the UK

The latest information on usage of contraception comes from the *General household survey 1993*.[2] Overall contraceptive uptake is 72% of women aged 16–49. This is a high figure when compared with many other countries.

Comparative use of the different methods is shown in Figure 2.1. Coitus interruptus (withdrawal) was still the most common method of birth control in the early twentieth century. In 1992 in my Bedfordshire

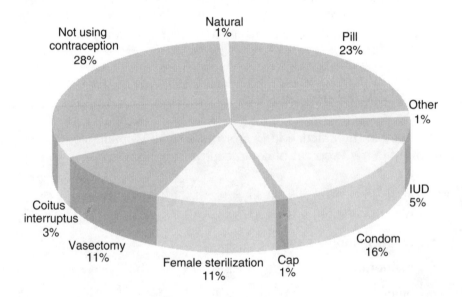

Figure 2.1: Current usage of different contraceptive methods by women aged 16–49 in Great Britain, 1993. 'Other' comprises injectables, spermicides and sponge (no longer available).

practice coitus interruptus had been used by 23% of women aged 20–49.[9]

The vulcanization of rubber in 1843 led to the replacement of skin condoms with latex condoms and the introduction of the Dutch cap in the mid-1880s. Coitus interruptus and condoms were the most commonly used methods until the introduction of the combined pill in 1961 and the progestogen-only pill in 1969. The pill became the most popular method of contraception, although during the 1980s usage dropped significantly. The reasons for this are not clear but may include the aftermath of pill scares, a rejection of artificial hormones in favour of more 'natural' methods and some individuals switching to condom use.

Over the last two decades there has been a dramatic rise in the popularity of sterilization, with as many as 55% of married or co-habiting women aged 40–44 using sterilization of themselves or their partner (*General household survey 1991* data). Since the mid-1980s there has been an increase in the uptake of condoms, probably resulting from the health education campaigns relating to the transmission of HIV. Since the pill first became available there has been a sevenfold reduction in oestrogen dose by the manufacturers. The popularity of female sterilization may well reflect the enormous social changes women have undergone in the last two decades: taking control of their lives, no longer having to cope with repeated unintended pregnancy, becoming a major part of the workforce, the rise of the 'career woman' and the phenomenon of voluntary childlessness.

The media

In the field of contraception the media have plenty of potential for doing enormous good. For instance, teenage magazines are read avidly and are a powerful source of information to supplement sex education given in schools and by parents. Women's magazines are a regular source of information on the choice of products available and the routes for obtaining them – medical or otherwise. They also exhort women to take more responsibility for their health – to attend health screening, where appropriate, and to lead healthier lives.

The problem is that the PHCT feels immediate pressure from any publicity, whether it be demand for methods not yet marketed or anxiety over a scare about their efficacy or safety.

At a more serious level, good news is seldom given the attention of bad news; and so 'bad news', for example, about the combined pill and either cancer or thromboembolism, has been given sensational headlines over the years by the press, TV and radio. The IUD, too, has received bad press largely due to assumptions by pressure groups and others that all devices are like the Dalkon Shield. More recently, Norplant has attracted a lot of unwarranted negative media attention; this may have been fuelled by a few solicitors keen on attracting personal injury cases.

Those who use contraceptives are very susceptible to the power of the media. In particular, consumers worry a lot about the safety of the combined pill. This anxiety, and the perceived side-effects from a method, are the commonest causes of switching method. Combine this with the notion that consumers choose their contraceptive as the least awful of the available range and we have a precarious state of affairs. Quite a lot of method switching goes on; a recent survey showed that one-fifth of women had been using their current or most recent method for less than a year.[5]

Pill scares

The two articles in the *Lancet* (22 October 1983) which preceded the 1983 'pill scare' gave rise to 34 articles in the national papers which took up 1339 column inches, and 161 articles in the provincial press taking up 4050 column inches.

The main failure of the press was to put the risks given into any sort of context with either numbers of extra cases of cancer or relative risk, and lack of mention of the beneficial effects of the pill to provide a balanced view. The Committee on Safety of Medicines (CSM) had not received an advance copy of the first paper and so could not give an assessment for the public or medical profession until later. The result was that many women panicked and stopped their pill. Figure 2.2 shows how the abortion rate rose after pill scares over the last 25 years. Preliminary figures show a 7% increase in abortion rates in the first quarter of 1996 compared with the same period in 1995.

There is some evidence that the same phenomenon occurred after the October 1995 venous thromboembolism scare. Here, although the CSM had sight of the unpublished papers, GPs had not been armed with the Committee's comments prior to the news breaking. A CSM

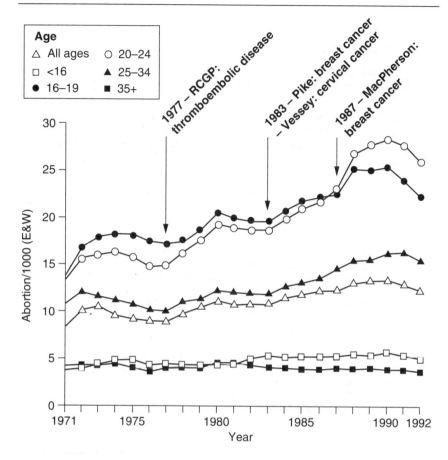

Figure 2.2: The effect of pill scares on abortion rates in 1977, 1983 and 1987. Reproduced with kind permission of the author and publisher.[10] Sadly my colleague David Bromham died on 3 December 1996.

mailing had been organized but the press conference had to be brought forward due to the information being leaked. Many emergency appointments were filled with anxious women but there was a lack of scientific information on which to base advice for them. Also, when the advice was forthcoming it was felt by many that it lacked practical relevance for doctors at the coalface because clinicians had not been consulted sufficiently. This particular pill scare was associated with a cluster of six research papers which appeared in the *Lancet* and the *BMJ* in December 1995 and January 1996. The two *BMJ* articles which attracted so many headlines were:

Third generation oral contraceptives and risk of myocardial infarction: an international case-control study

Michael A Lewis, Walter O Spitzer, Lothar A J Heinemann, Kenneth D MacRae, Rudolf Bruppacher, Margaret Thorogood on behalf of Transnational Research Group on Oral Contraceptives and the Health of Young Women

Abstract

Objective—To test whether use of combined oral contraceptives containing third generation progestogens is associated with altered risk of myocardial infarction.

to 6·3) (P=0·003) for use of second generation products v no current use and 1·1 (0·4 to 3·4) (P=0·9) for use of third generation products v no current use. Among the confounding variables the independent contribution of smoking (for which adjustment was

BMJ   VOLUME 312   13 JANUARY 1996

Third generation oral contraceptives and risk of venous thromboembolic disorders: an international case-control study

Walter O Spitzer, Michael A Lewis, Lothar A J Heinemann, Margaret Thorogood, Kenneth D MacRae on behalf of Transnational Research Group on Oral Contraceptives and the Health of Young Women

Abstract

Objective—To test whether use of combined oral contraceptives containing third generation progestogens is associated with altered risk of venous thromboembolism.

contraceptives and have concluded that their risks are balanced by benefits.[1-4] Since their introduction, oral contraceptives have undergone considerable development intended to reduce the risk of adverse effects. In the 1970s second generation drugs were introduced

BMJ   VOLUME 312   13 JANUARY 1996

In contrast, in June 1996 a *Lancet* paper on breast cancer and the pill had already been processed by the CSM due to wise cooperation of the journal's editor, and a statement came down the fax cascade to GPs prior to publication. This paper caused minimal comment in the media and the better collaboration between authors, journal and CSM was surely a major factor in this.

What all this means for the future is uncertain. Pill scares will undoubtedly occur in the future; hopefully there will be more warning time, and more consultation and control over the way in which

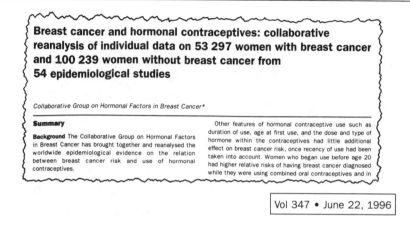

Breast cancer and hormonal contraceptives: collaborative reanalysis of individual data on 53 297 women with breast cancer and 100 239 women without breast cancer from 54 epidemiological studies

Collaborative Group on Hormonal Factors in Breast Cancer*

Summary

Background The Collaborative Group on Hormonal Factors in Breast Cancer has brought together and reanalysed the worldwide epidemiological evidence on the relation between breast cancer risk and use of hormonal contraceptives.

Other features of hormonal contraceptive use such as duration of use, age at first use, and the dose and type of hormone within the contraceptives had little additional effect on breast cancer risk, once recency of use had been taken into account. Women who began use before age 20 had higher relative risks of having breast cancer diagnosed while they were using combined oral contraceptives and in

Vol 347 • June 22, 1996

the information is released. It pays to be forearmed as well as fore-warned, for example, by agreeing a protocol for a practice helpline to be set up if the need ever arises. Another approach is to explain to each patient the nature of ongoing studies on drugs that are pre-scribed, and exactly what to do if they read of or hear anything that causes anxiety. 'Crisis management', as this is called, is a key part of the practice business plan – see Chapter 8.

Abortion – trends

Since the introduction of legal abortion in Great Britain in 1968, abortion rates have steadily risen, apart from gentle falls in the late 1970s and early 1980s and a current fall since 1990. The abortion rate gives us some idea of the extent of unplanned pregnancy.

Factors that influence the abortion rate are:

- changing fertility patterns
- changing age structure of women of childbearing age
- changing contraceptive use
- changing attitudes to abortion
- prevailing economic climate.

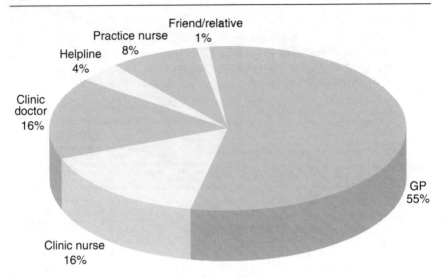

Figure 2.3: Contraceptive Education Service Survey, UK, 1995, women aged 16–49. Women were asked 'Who would you prefer to talk to if you had any difficulties using any contraceptive method?'[5]

Possibly up to half of all pregnancies are to some extent unintended. About one in five pregnancies are terminated (one in two in the under-16s and over-40s).

Figure 2.3 shows the results of interviews of women aged 16–49, responding to a question about who they would prefer to talk to if they had any difficulties using any contraceptive method. Members of the PHCT come out way ahead! Rather surprisingly, practice nurses are not as popular as one would guess.

Summary

In Chapters 1 and 2, I have attempted to provide a public health and a general practice perspective for the delivery of family planning services in the late 1990s. The rest of this book is very practical and focuses on how a good family planning service in general practice should be run. It covers some topics never before included in family planning texts, and pulls together quite disparate strands of information relating to the management of a good service.

How to set up a family planning service in general practice

Regulations

The regulations governing the provision of a contraceptive service within general practice are surprisingly few. No previous training is required of the GPs and nurses providing the service. This is in marked contrast to the trust clinic service where trusts will not employ staff without post-registration qualifications in family planning.

Any GP principal may apply to the health authority to be placed on the contraceptive list and is automatically added. This is unlike child health surveillance, the obstetric list and minor surgery where previous experience is essential. Contraceptive services are supplied by 98% of GPs.

In addition, with the advent of the new claim forms (see below) GPs are no longer required to certify that 'they have had regard to and been guided by modern authoritative medical opinion such as the advice given by the Standing Medical Advisory Committee in the *Handbook of contraceptive practice*'.[11] This is no bad thing as the booklet in question is out of date and not due to be revised. (Confusingly, the *Red Book* [paragraph 29.6] still claims that they do!)

The fact that the regulations do not specify any quality standard is no excuse for providing a substandard service. Training, qualifications and updating are all requirements of modern day practice and these are covered in Chapter 9.

Guidelines

Currently, very few practices have guidelines and there are no national guidelines on family planning. Guidelines for doctors on emergency contraception drawn up by the Faculty of Family Planning and Reproductive Health Care were included in the emergency contraception information pack issued to all GPs by the Contraceptive

Education Service in 1995. However, these guidelines were not drawn up in the strict scientific and multidisciplinary way mentioned in Chapter 9.

It is hoped national guidelines will be developed in the future and local protocols can be adapted from these. As this book is written the Royal College of Obstetricians and Gynaecologists is drawing up guidelines on female sterilization, vasectomy and induced abortion. Further remarks are made about guidelines in Chapter 9.

Women's choice of service

As explained in Chapter 2, in my practice 41% of women seek contraceptive advice outside the practice. Women who choose the combined pill, women in their family-building years and those who are married or in stable relationships are particularly likely to choose a general practice family planning service. Others may choose to go elsewhere.

It is important to remember that the Government continues to support a dual provision of family planning outlet[12-16] and the trust clinics complement the GP service. It is vital that the PHCT does not try to recruit reluctant individuals to use its service. Some patients feel they cannot go to their GP. The reasons for this may be complex but are often due to a reluctance to admit to sexual desires, problems or fantasies. Some people cannot discuss this part of themselves, with the associated feeling of vulnerability, in front of the doctor on whom they rely when they are ill, or who is well known by their family. Any attempt on the part of the GP to provide for every need in this area is likely to fail. Practice nurses may face the same problems in the patients they see, though those patients who find it hard to talk to their doctor may find it easier to talk to the practice nurse.

Young people

Catering for the needs of young people is a problem. It has been said that GPs are generally seen as inappropriate sources of help, for various reasons, by both young people who have and those who have not approached their family doctor.[17]

Ideally, young persons' centres should be situated away from premises run according to a medical model. Strategies to make services more accessible to young people need to take account of major constraints on young people's ability to travel – lack of money to pay for transport and limited geographical knowledge. Some of the key features of an ideal young persons' centre are:

- open more than once a week – Saturday and Monday opening a minimum

- open between 3.30 p.m. and 8 p.m.

- drop-in arrangements with some appointments too

- qualified counsellor available

- a relaxed and informal environment

- all staff given initial and ongoing support

- publicity in schools, colleges, youth clubs, sports and leisure centres, night clubs and public places.

To provide such a service in a surgery is a challenge to say the least and possibly inappropriate. Brook Advisory Centres meet these criteria but are available in only a few parts of the UK. Some practices seem to have had a good go at setting up a service for young people: six are mentioned in a Health Education Authority compendium.[18]

There are two main ways of making contact with teenagers – normally a healthy group and infrequent attenders at the surgery. The first is by invitation on reaching the age of 13, 14, 15 or 16. Parental consent has been obtained for the younger teenagers by the PHCTs who have attempted this method – which in itself creates a barrier. A health check can be offered which includes measurement of weight, height and blood pressure, discussion of diet, smoking, alcohol and drugs, and contraception as appropriate. One practice which invited 15-year-olds gave the pre-school-leaving immunization too, but found that many teenagers were accompanied by their parents!

Responses are variable but can be encouraging. A study in Birmingham[19] showed parental refusal to be uncommon, and attendance rates were around 50% for girls and 30% for boys.

The second way is a drop-in facility on a Saturday morning from 11 a.m. to 1 p.m. This has been tried in several areas. There is a concern amongst the teenagers that they might bump into family members at the surgery. The uptake amongst boys can be poor.[20] There is a problem too with publicity. Material can be sent to those on the practice list but many of those attending are from other practices. News travels very much by word of mouth. Formal publicity in the places mentioned previously for a practice-based service is not possible.[21]

Plans for a drop-in service should be made with the local trust family planning service and local youth workers according to the principles outlined in Chapter 1.

A dedicated clinic?

The family planning service may be provided in ordinary surgery appointments with doctors and nurses, or in a combination of ordinary surgery appointments plus a dedicated clinic run by a member of the PHCT with a special interest. Consideration should be given as to whether a dedicated clinic will extend beyond or be run entirely outside normal surgery hours. A further additional service is to have a practice nurse run a drop-in session without appointments.

A point to make here is that the contribution of a dedicated clinic to raising standards throughout a practice is severely limited. Such a clinic may be useful for carrying out specialized procedures such as IUD/IUS and subdermal implant insertion and removal but the vast majority of pill checks and other routine work will take place in ordinary surgeries and so all members of the PHCT will need to adopt protocols if particular policies and standards of care are to be adhered to.

Whatever decision is made, opportunistic discussion of family planning will take place during all sorts of consultations. This must be recognized and built upon, especially for infrequent or reluctant attenders.

Although it is not feasible to deliver a service solely through a dedicated clinic, it is beneficial if one GP and/or nurse take a lead role in setting up and running the service. They can pioneer the protocols, be a point of contact for outside agencies, offer specialized advice to the practice and accept internal referrals.

Premises and equipment

Furniture, fittings and layout

There are no requirements for premises in general practice specific to family planning. There are minimum requirements for practices generally and for minor surgery. Secure and comfortable changing facilities for women and curtains around couches to ensure privacy are essential. Toys can be provided in the waiting room for accompanying children, but these now have to be cleaned in accordance with health and safety regulations. Remarkably small details can enable patients to feel their requirements have been well thought out – something as simple as a hook and coat-hanger for clothes, or – on the educational side – a well-stocked display of free, up-to-date educational leaflets, such as the FPA's Contraceptive Education Service (CES) leaflets. Some of these facilities are essential, and some are to be recommended, but all in all they can have a powerful effect on the image the practice presents to patients in its catchment area.

Instruments/equipment

It is beyond the scope of this book to list all instruments needed for family planning practice. Training courses on intrauterine techniques and subdermal implants will provide all the information that is needed.

It is worth mentioning autoclaves here. These must comply with the European Union (EU) and British Standards. The Medical Devices Agency of the DOH ensures compliance with these standards. Wrapped instruments are very convenient; they remain sterile in their pouches. This is helpful when procedures need to be undertaken at short notice and there is no time to preplan. However, only certain autoclaves are designed to sterilize wrapped instruments: the Prestige Medical Century 2100, the SES Vacuum Little Sister 3 and the SES 2000 are examples.

Readers who require further information on the technical aspects of sterilization should refer to Health Technical Memorandum 2010 Part 1: *Management Policy, Sterilization*, NHS Estates, HMSO, London, 1994. Preventative maintenance is required quarterly with an additional annual check by a sterilizer engineer.

The range of choice of method offered to women impacts on the equipment needed. Ideally all contraceptive methods should be offered, but to provide condoms is not always easy (see Chapter 10).

Consumables

Very few consumables are needed. Same-day pregnancy testing is the main service that must be offered. It is an expense against which no financial claim can be made to the health authority. Rapid pregnancy testing is particularly important nowadays with the advent of medical terminations that must be performed before 9 weeks' gestation. Many hospital laboratories cut back long ago on pregnancy testing to decrease their departmental expenditure.

It is not permissible to charge patients for tests; pregnancy testing is regarded as treatment and to charge would be a breach of paragraph 32 of a GP's Terms of Service.[22] Neither is it acceptable to send unwilling patients to the chemist for a test to be performed by the pharmacist or for the patient to purchase a home test. Bulk-buying of test kits by the practice reduces unit costs, although expiry dates will need to be taken into account. Note that many women who suspect they may be pregnant will already have done a home test.

Choice of method offered

Choice of method offered by the practice should be as wide as possible. The following two groups of parameters affect the couple's choice, and importantly, may give some insight into how the choice is best presented (see also Method teaching, p.23).

Personal choice is dependent partly on the method itself, namely:

• efficacy

• availability

• cost (if not available on the NHS).

Choice is also dependent on the attitudes and knowledge of the individual:

• acceptability of method

- ease of use

- influences of friends/relatives

- personal circumstances, such as career/employment status, financial status

- social circumstances

- circumstances of sexual relationship (e.g. number of partners, length of relationship, involvement of partner in choice)

- phase of family-building (delayers, spacers or stoppers), or preference for not having a family

- age

- religion

- culture

- risk of sexually transmitted infection

- perceived side effects.

Monitoring of patients

Monitoring intervals for the different methods should be laid down in the family planning protocols for your practice, as should the procedures carried out at each visit. As far as possible these protocols should be evidence-based (see Chapter 9).

Method teaching

Users need to be told and shown how to use their method. An understanding of how the method works decreases user failure. Method teaching is vital both at the first consultation and as reinforcement as a method is selected and used; nurses are particularly useful in both instances. For women to make an informed choice of method, resources such as demonstration packs of pills, models, on-screen computer programs or videos should be used, always backed up with written material.

The following leaflets are produced by the CES (Figure 3.1). All of them have been subject to scrutiny by the Plain English Campaign and, where appropriate, awarded a Crystal Mark. All leaflets produced are consumer-tested. Leaflets are dated, and updated when new information becomes available.

- Your guide to contraception (also available in Bengali, Gujarati, Hindi, Punjabi, Urdu)
- The combined pill
- The progestogen-only pill
- Injections and implants
- The IUD
- The IUS
- Diaphragms and caps
- The male and female condom
- Natural methods
- Male and female sterilization
- After you've had your baby – contraceptive choices
- Emergency contraception
- Your guide to safer sex and the condom
- A guide to family planning services
- 4 Boys
- 4 Girls
- Is everybody doing it?
- Periods

There is some evidence that patients advised to discontinue the pill are less likely to be provided with an alternative method by GPs than by family planning clinics.[23] Knowledge of certain aspects of contraception is not so good among GPs.[24] Women taught pill-taking rules by GPs appear to remember them less accurately than those who are taught in clinics.[25,26] Finally, patients requesting termination of pregnancy have been shown to have poorer knowledge of contraception

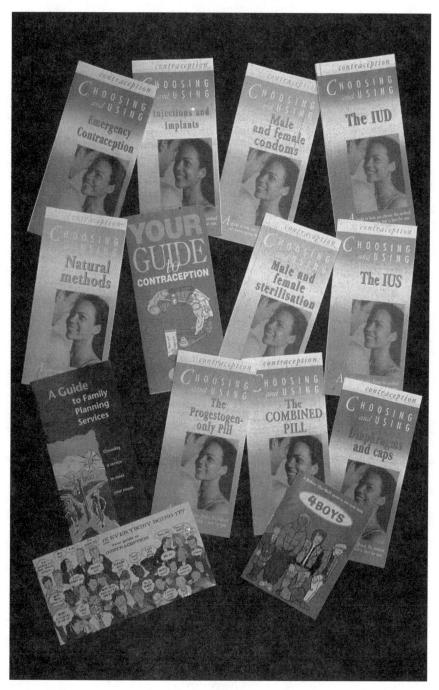

Figure 3.1: Examples of current Contraceptive Education Service leaflets.

when their source of advice was their GP in some studies[27] but not in others.[28]

It is regrettable – to say the least – if health professionals contribute towards the failure of a patient's method. Careful consideration of the resource material and structure of method teaching used in the consultation should remove the differences that exist between general practice and trust clinics.

Claim forms and fees

The Government's *Patients Not Paper: Fewer Better Forms* initiative in England and Wales culminated in the demise of the oft-quoted FP1001, FP1002 and FP1003 forms in July 1996.

The equivalent forms in Scotland were GP102, GP103 and GP104, and in Northern Ireland still are FP1001, FP1002 and FP1003 (but of different design).

In England and Wales the first two forms (FP1001 and FP1002) are now encompassed by the item of service multiclaim form GMS4 (Figure 3.2). The third form for temporary residents (FP1003) is covered by the GMS3. To sighs of relief all round the patient no longer has to sign the form so that a claim can be made when it is realized the patient has left the building!

Scotland has the advantage of an item of service multiclaim form (GPC) for the ordinary contraceptive fee, IUD fitting fee and temporary resident contraceptive fee. This came into effect on 1 April 1996.

In Northern Ireland a multiclaim form (MULTI1) is planned to supersede FP1001 and FP1002 some time during 1997.

The old bureaucratic system of checking all fee claims before payment has been replaced by post-payment verification. Practice records must be kept of what has been claimed as the signature on the form certifies that an audit trail is available at the practice for inspection.

Claims must not be made for advising a man on his own. Any woman, irrespective of whether or not she is registered for general medical services, may apply to receive contraceptive services. Claims may be made for advising a woman to seek specialist contraceptive help elsewhere in the NHS, for fitting of a cap or after a failed IUD insertion.

Insertion or reinsertion of an IUD attracts a higher fee for a period of 1 year. Health authorities pay IUD fees quarterly – the lower fee in

NHS

Item of service multi-claim

GMS4

Please tick only one box ☑ then complete in BLOCK CAPITALS

- ☐ Registration examination
- ☐ Night consultation
- ☐ Vaccination & immunisations
- ☐ Contraceptive services
- ☐ Minor surgery
- ☐ Anaesthetic
- ☐ Dental haemorrhage

	Date	Patient's name	Date of birth	NHS number	A	B	HA	Notes
1								
2								
3								
4								
5								
6								
7								
8								
9								
10								

I declare to the best of my belief that this information is correct and I claim the appropriate payment as set out in the Statement of Fees and Allowances. An audit trail is available at the practice for inspection by the HA's authorised officers and auditors appointed by the Audit Commission.

Authorised signature

Name   Date

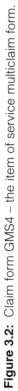

Practice stamp

Figure 3.2: Claim form GMS4 – the item of service multiclaim form.

equal instalments, the higher fee with a higher rate first instalment to reflect the additional work involved in fitting a device.

NHS item of service contraception fees as at April 1996 are:

Ordinary fee	£14.25 p.a.
IUD fee	£47.70
(1st quarter	£36.90
2nd quarter	£3.60
3rd quarter	£3.60
4th quarter	£3.60)
Temporary resident fee	£3.56 (up to 3 months)
Temporary resident IUD fitting	£23.85.

Insertion and removal of an implantable device, and vasectomy, attract no fee as these operations do not appear on the list of minor surgical procedures. Item of service claims are made annually, but must not be sent in at under 11 months or after 18 months if the payment is to be continuous.

Abortion

Abortion is an integral part of birth control provision. Objectives of the service, from a general practice perspective, should include:

• minimal delay in the referral system in order to reduce levels of second-trimester termination (operation to be performed within 2–5 days of the patient making a firm decision)

• 95% of abortions should be provided by the NHS.

Fundholders are likely to have more control over the above than non-fundholders.

Recall

It is usual to rely on those needing further supplies of pills and those using diaphragms/caps to arrange to book themselves in for follow-up. A much better system is to develop practice computer codes which can be recorded at each check.

For the pill, the patient can be asked whether she intends to continue the pill or to stop in the near future. One of two codes is entered at the time of the consultation. Monthly recall date reports are run on claims made 12 months previously and claims can be renewed for those with the 'intends to continue pill' code entered at the last visit.

It is best to have all those on injectables on a recall system since overdue injections are troublesome for both staff and patient alike. A weekly report is best for injectable recall so that a telephone reminder can be made. It can be more difficult for those not on the telephone; a letter or a visit to the house may be necessary. The author's most challenging problem with injectable recall was a forgetful patient living in a tent on a friend's lawn!

For IUDs, the IUS and for implantables, recall is necessary so that annual checks get done and patients are not lost to follow-up. Computerized tracking is recommended and outlined in Chapter 7. Those with long-acting methods *in situ* should come up on monthly reports at 3 months after fitting and on each anniversary from fitting. Predefined reminder letters can then be sent out. Some patients will choose not to attend for a follow-up if they have no symptoms and are happy to continue with the method.

Certain patients come to rely on the recall telephone call while others find the reminder reassuring although they have remembered to make their appointment.

It is important to discuss recall with patients to ensure they are comfortable with the systems used. Telephone calls raise confidentiality issues when a third party answers the telephone.

Publicity

Publicity for the family planning service is important and contributes to the perceived value of the service (existing patients) as well as its level of uptake (new patients). Not only should there be an entry in the practice leaflet, but posters should be placed in the surgery waiting room.

Improvements in the service should be announced in the practice newsletter or by a poster in the waiting room.

A resources/health promotion room on the premises with books, leaflets and reference files for patients to browse through is valuable, as long as patients know that it exists and materials are of good quality, up to date and well presented.

Publicity material needs to convey these key items of information:

* who provides the service

* what services are available

* where services are available

* when services are available

* that services are:

   – private and confidential

   – free.

Expanding and improving the service

A decision can be made to offer the family planning service to women outside the practice, registering them for contraceptive services only. Some neighbouring practices may regard this as tantamount to poaching as the patient concerned might switch practices if suitably impressed. But in these days of the market economy people should be free to choose the service they prefer and services should be free to market themselves. A distinction must be made between this type of service expansion and the coercion of unwilling patients, who for very good reasons of their own may prefer to go outside the practice – see p. 18. (Of course, your own patients may choose to go to another GP for contraception.)

A service should be sensitive to the needs of people of different races, cultures, ages and religions. Men should not be forgotten. Education, information and advice should be offered. Accessibility, convenience, confidentiality and anonymity have been identified as key determinants of service use. Consumers on the whole tend to prefer a less 'medicalized' service.

Financial aspects

There has been widespread misunderstanding about the contraceptive fees claimed by GPs. There have been assertions in the medical press that general practice family planning services are more expensive to the tax payer than trust clinics and that practices can earn ever increasing amounts of money. This really is pie in the sky. A review of the economics of family planning[6] showed that the cost per attender is relatively low for all forms of provision.

While it is true that the cost of dispensing contraceptives on FP10s is greater than the cost of supplies bought in bulk for clinics, usually no additional manpower is needed to run the GP service and the cost of premises and equipment is absorbed into the practice as a whole.

The fundamental concept many fail to appreciate is that payment of item-of-service fees to GPs costs the Treasury nothing. Each year since 1960 the Review Body on Doctors' and Dentists' Pay has recommended what it considers to be an appropriate level of net (without expenses element) income for GPs and the Government decides the average level of income for all GPs.

From this cash sum is paid capitation fees, basic allowances, item-of-service fees and so on. By doing more contraceptive work, a GP will earn more for his/her practice compared with a GP not doing so much, and more than the average income set by the Government. However, the extra cash earned will come off the amount earned by other GPs; it is not extra cash produced at the Treasury. If the global cash sum allotted to contraceptive services were to be exceeded then the excess would be clawed back from the following year's global cash sum and the fees reduced.

Despite the above comments it does pay to be meticulous in claiming for contraceptive services, particularly in filling in claim forms promptly and submitting them at the appropriate time, and in constantly trying to expand and improve the service in the way described earlier in the chapter.

It has been estimated that the average GP claimed £1883 for contraceptive services in 1995–6. Income per patient for the year-end March 1996 was as follows:

England	100.1p
Wales	97.6p
Scotland	88.6p
Northern Ireland	79.0p.

It is likely that the introduction of the multiclaim forms will increase the potential for income from contraceptive services because sometimes there may have been embarrassment at asking patients to sign the old forms. However, as already mentioned, there will not be an income bonanza for practices because of the limitation of cash allotted for contraceptive services within the NHS.

4

The role of the practice nurse

Shelley Mehigan and Catriona Sutherland

The development of practice nursing

Practice nursing has changed beyond recognition since the 1970s when it evolved from treatment-room nursing. As the value of having a surgery-based nurse became recognized and more GPs became aware of this, the role developed in a number of ways. Individual surgeries and GPs identified the needs and tasks that they felt were appropriate to them and, as often happens with a new specialty, initially the role varied greatly.

At this time nurses brought the skills they had already learned from the various hospital and community settings they had worked in, and were taught new skills by the doctors who employed them according to the needs of that practice. Thus there were many nurses across the country who had a wide variety of skills. Some of them felt isolated but, with time, practice nurses have joined together to share their experiences and this has given rise to a number of local and national professional groups.

The Practice Nurse Association is now the largest single professional group within the Royal College of Nursing (RCN). Likewise, as the role has evolved, training needs have been identified which have led to a number of courses being developed in specific areas like asthma, diabetes, immunization and venepuncture. Colleges and universities have started offering practice nurse courses at diploma and degree level.

Family planning courses predate practice nursing but recently have been accessed by more practice nurses than other groups. Family planning has been identified as a specialty particularly appropriate for practice nurses to train in.

Underused and undervalued

A recent survey by the Contraceptive Education Service[5] showed that only 1% of women thought about discussing a choice or change of contraception with practice nurses and that only 4% would choose to seek advice from a practice nurse if she needed a change of method.

This is disappointing and it seems likely that this is because people do not know that their practice nurse may be trained in this specialty. Perhaps general practices are not very good at promoting the fact that this is a service that a particular nurse can provide. Unless a dedicated family planning session is run then the fact that a nurse is able to provide this service needs to be advertised.

It sometimes seems that patients become aware of services by accident when attending for other more obvious ones like holiday immunization or if they have been referred by the GP. This may be because nurses have tended to pick up skills in a fairly haphazard way, particularly when training has been in-service. In the same way they may attend study days to extend, improve or update their original training.

In the past practice nurses were seen as only working in the 'treatment room' and it may have been assumed that they were only able to do dressings or take blood pressures. Many people are unaware of how the role has changed and developed over the years and how some nurses have become very experienced practitioners in certain areas. *This attitude is true of some doctors as well as patients.* Whereas some patients may simply be unaware of the skills that have been learned, doctors have often chosen to ignore them. In the past some doctors may have felt that nurses developing advanced skills would encroach on their own areas of expertise and have resisted this. However, as the role has become established and recognized the advantages have become apparent and doctors are appreciating that this enables them to concentrate on other areas which are outside nurses' experience or competence and this can increase their own job satisfaction as well as providing a more efficient service for patients. The fault has often rested with nurses themselves who have been unable to assert themselves and negotiate with the other members of the PHCT as to the extent of their skills. As practice nursing has spread with support from the profession, nurses have become better at communicating their expertise.

Accessibility

The practice nurse is now becoming recognized as an accessible health professional by patients, GPs and other team members. Many patients see nurses as being 'less busy' than doctors and possibly more accommodating, since some nurses are able to build a few additional slots into their more flexible appointment schedules. Patients are quick to work out who is the appropriate person to consult for a particular problem, realizing that requiring a cervical smear or contraception need not be a 'medical' problem that requires access to a doctor.

Patients may choose to consult the practice nurse about family planning and related matters for a number of reasons. These may be:

- the nurse is a female

- the nurse is known to the woman because she has carried out her children's immunizations, etc.

- the woman may 'try out' the nurse with a problem, asking if it is something she should 'see the doctor about'

- some patients prefer to discuss their problems with a nurse, feeling that the nurse is less threatening than the doctor

- other team members may suggest to the woman that the nurse is the appropriate person to see.

Young people

All patients need and deserve a high quality, accessible and confidential family planning service. This is particularly so of young people, who will not use a service unless it meets their specific requirements. The timing of sessions is important with after-school being a favoured time.[29] Using the family planning services in general practice can be very discreet since the young person may appear to be attending for a consultation about her acne, periods or an ingrowing toenail!

Young people especially may be more likely to see the practice nurse as someone who appears to be less threatening than a doctor, particularly at a first visit when they may be testing out the service. The receptionist is important here as the welcome young people receive when they attend will directly influence how they use this and other services in the practice (see Chapter 5).

Misunderstandings about issues of confidentiality among young people and any PHCT members need to be identified and challenged, otherwise they will be perpetuated (see Chapter 12).

It is not unusual for a young woman to attend her consultation supported by 'my friend'. This may lead to a crowded consulting room but is an ideal opportunity to dispel fear, to spread information to a wider audience and to encourage future attendances. Word of mouth is an excellent source of referral.

Education

Nurse education has changed, over recent years in particular, at pre- and post-registration level. New courses are being developed all the time. Family planning, contraception and women's health are specific areas where excellent courses are available. The four National Boards for Nursing, Midwifery and Health Visiting currently approve the following courses:

English National Board 901

Welsh National Board 901 Family Planning in Society

Scottish National Board Family Planning Course

Northern Ireland National Board Family Planning Nursing Course.

These are post-registration courses open to nurses holding a first-level registration on the United Kingdom Central Council (UKCC) Professional Register. They offer training to participants on giving advice, counselling and competent care to people of all ages in matters relating to fertility and its control, sexuality and health screening. Courses are part time and based on a minimum of 12 study days and 12 clinical sessions in approved training placements, completed over a period of 20 weeks.

These courses are more comprehensive than the Diploma of the Faculty of Family Planning (DFFP) for doctors! It has been shown that few practice nurses hold this qualification and many would like training and are on waiting lists for places.[30,31] One reason why there is an apparent shortage of places is the necessity to provide clinical placements, and as clinics and clinic sessions have been cut this has become increasingly difficult.

The problem is being addressed in a number of parts of the UK by using appropriately trained practice nurses (i.e. those with a family planning qualification, experience and a teaching certificate) to offer clinical training in general practice. This has happened in a number of areas for some time as the value of training in a variety of settings has been recognized. As more practice nurses become trained this will develop further.

Currently these courses are being run in different ways by different educational establishments with many being split into two modules providing either an introduction to the subject or the theory in the first module and more in-depth knowledge and clinical practice in the second. This has the advantage for those nurses who require only a basic understanding of the subject to undertake the first module, whereas those who need to be competent in clinical care or who wish to specialize in the field must complete both modules.

It is probably impracticable, too costly and unnecessary for *all* practice nurses to undertake full family planning training. However, note should be taken of the English National Board guidance[32] relating to this which states that 'Those nurses responsible for direct care in the family planning service within general practice must undertake the full course'. It goes on to say that nurses working in general practice responsible for answering general queries must undertake the most appropriate module to meet their needs.

Informal in-service training by GPs in family planning is not acceptable. Some colleges and health authorities run 'Introduction to family planning' courses and study days which can be very useful for providing a basic knowledge and understanding of contraceptive methods. Access to these different levels of training allows flexibility in the provision of family planning care.

The English National Board has also approved the A08 Advanced Family Planning Nursing Course. Open to experienced family planning nurses this course allows for further, more advanced and in-depth training in wider issues relating to sexual health. Psychosexual seminar work is an important component. Currently this also includes learning pelvic bimanual and breast examination but not for routine screening (see p. 77). Some nurses who have completed this course have had further training in more specialist areas, for example, fitting and removal of Norplant, fitting of IUDs and psychosexual counselling as well as becoming nurse specialists in a number of other related areas such as the menopause.

Role development

A nurse who has completed a full family planning course can, with suitable experience and, if necessary, further training, develop her role in a number of ways. Many nurses may be expected to undertake cervical smears and this may require further training since not all family planning training courses include this to a high enough level of competence.

A trained and experienced nurse is able to provide information, advice and support to patients on a wide range of related topics. Although many of these are outside the scope of this book, they may include:

- vaginal health and infections
- menstrual problems
- preconception care
- contraception
- breast awareness
- cervical cytology
- fertility problems
- sexual anxieties
- rape/sexual abuse
- relationship difficulties
- eating disorders
- adolescent development
- the menopause
- lifestyle.

Pill checks

This is a much misused term and is used by some practices to indicate that a patient merely needs her blood pressure taken before a further supply of pills may be issued. However, if a nurse undertakes to do this she is accepting a certain level of responsibility for the patient's wellbeing and is accountable for her actions. She may leave herself open to disciplinary action if it later transpires that it was inappropriate at that time for the patient to continue with the medication, or if she was working outside the UKCC Code of Professional Conduct.

Nurse reissuing of contraceptives

The Crown Report[33] recommended that the prescription of contraceptives by appropriately trained nurses should be considered separately from nurse prescribing in general but this has not happened. The Prescribing by Nurses Act 1992 made prescribing by nurses legal but a subsequent amendment restricted its relevance to certain groups that did not include family planning nurses.

Once the practice nurse has consolidated her family planning training with some experience and feels confident, it may be appropriate for her to reissue prescriptions of previously prescribed, ongoing contraception using protocols. These will need to be negotiated with one or more of her GPs and will need to include which contraceptives may be issued, what is to be checked at each visit and criteria for referral to the doctor.

Protocols should be written and signed by both the responsible doctor and any individual nurse to whom it applies. These may be used for oral contraception and for injectables (see Appendix 2). In the case of oral contraceptives the FP10 must be signed by a doctor before the nurse may issue the prescription. The use of protocols for initial prescribing is under debate with differing legal interpretations of the Medicines Act 1968. It is acceptable for protocols to be used by appropriately trained family planning nurses for providing supplies of hormonal contraceptives, where the initial assessment and prescription has been made by a doctor and a prescription covering further supplies has been completed and signed by the doctor, either at the time of the consultation or in advance of anticipated follow-up visits. Under no circumstances should a nurse accept a signed blank FP10 from a GP.

For drop-in sessions another system will need to be used. For example, patients can be asked to return if they do not need their supply immediately or they can wait in the surgery until the nurse can see the doctor to get an FP10 signed.

The RCN has published guidelines for nurses undertaking family planning in general practice in its *Issues in nursing and health* series.[34]

In the case of injectables it may be that a supply of these is kept in the surgery and dispensed directly or a patient may be given an FP10 for her next supply at each visit. These can then be administered by the nurse using the protocol.

A system must also be in place for the nurse to be able to access the doctor in case of queries and problems which need to be dealt with at that time.

Telephone advice

Allocating time to respond to queries and problems on the telephone can be a very useful way of dealing with anxiety among patients and can reduce the demand for unnecessary appointments. Ideally it is best if a time can be set aside on a regular basis when the nurse can take telephone calls, for example, either before or after her surgery session. This means the service can be actively promoted to ensure it is fully utilized (see Pill scares, p. 12). The availability of telephone advice can be publicized in the practice leaflet or by a poster in the waiting area and by telling people who attend family planning appointments.

As with all other aspects of family planning provision in general practice telephone advice should only be given by a nurse who has had some training in family planning as she would be working outside her professional code of conduct (see p. 44) if she undertook duties that she was not competent to provide.

If patients ring for advice when the nurse is not available to give advice, they can be asked to call back, the nurse can call them back, or they can ring a helpline such as the Contraceptive Education Service (CES).

Emergency contraception

This is a particular area where it may be appropriate for a trained practice nurse to give advice and help.

By its nature emergency contraception is required at short notice and it may be difficult for some patients to access it within the time limit. This is where teamwork can be especially important. The receptionist is of paramount importance as the person who deals with requests for appointments (see p. 47). In the case of emergency contraception, requests may be disguised in some way as people may be too embarrassed to explain why they need an urgent appointment. Receptionists need to be sensitive to these requests and able to direct patients to an appropriate member of the team without asking intrusive questions, which takes skill and understanding. It may be possible for patients to be fitted in with the practice nurse to discuss their needs.

The practice nurse who has some training in and knowledge of contraception can then assess the need in any particular case. She can take an accurate history which is vital in deciding if emergency contraception is necessary or appropriate, for example, to exclude someone who misunderstands its use and may already be pregnant. Having decided that it is necessary the nurse can then refer to whichever doctor is available or a doctor who has been designated as responsible for emergency contraception at any given time. The use of a protocol agreed jointly by nurse and GP for managing emergency contraception clarifies the role of the nurse and is strongly recommended.

Counselling

Counselling and information-giving play an important part in the field of family planning as in many other areas of medicine. Nurses develop a number of skills throughout their training and the ability to listen is one of these. Counselling in a formal way requires further training but there are many instances in every day practice where the ability to listen is invaluable. Family planning courses include specific aspects of counselling, for example, in relation to preconception, subfertility and pre- and post-termination. The advanced training includes seminar work in psychosexual counselling.

Counselling is time-consuming, and is quite different from information and advice-giving, but it is an area which can be very valuable and rewarding and it is something which nurses can do particularly well. They are often perceived as being more approachable and having more time than doctors in general. In a busy general practice session the nurse may need to allocate separate appointment times for counselling and it is often appropriate to ask patients to return at another time to discuss difficult problems.

Female barrier methods

The experienced nurse is usually the best person to teach the use of female barrier methods, this being an area in which nurses tend to excel. A comprehensive 'cap teach' can take as long as 30 minutes, and nurses can more easily build an appointment of this length into their schedules. It is essential that 'protected' time is available for the teaching of female barrier methods. This will help to prevent user failure and make women more likely to persevere with the method.

The practice nurse as a resource

The practice nurse may be key to the access to resources necessary to the family planning service. The resources may be:

- information leaflets (usually available from the health promotion unit); plus leaflets about related health promotion topics, e.g. breast awareness

- information about specialist agencies (see p. 119) – Endometriosis Society, Miscarriage Association, BACUP, Rape Crisis, Eating Disorders Association, etc.

- pharmaceutical representatives – liaising as to the availability of leaflets, posters, teaching aids etc.

- the fact that the nurse works in other family planning settings and is a member of professional groups and organizations.

Teamwork

The provision of a comprehensive family planning service is entirely dependent on good teamwork. In general practice the team may be large and include doctors, nurses, receptionists, health visitors, midwives, continence advisers, counsellors, etc. Patients benefit from the team members understanding and appreciating each other's roles, skills and expertise. This will ensure the best care for the patient from the most appropriate member of the team.

In addition, there should be an awareness of the services available outside the practice to which it may be appropriate to refer a patient. These services may include: young persons' clinics, specialist family planning clinics (e.g. for 'lost IUD threads'), termination counselling, psychosexual counselling, genitourinary medicine clinics, colposcopy, sterilization and genetic counselling (see also Chapter 6).

Confidentiality

Every patient, regardless of age or circumstance, is entitled to complete confidentiality. This duty of confidentiality is owed by all members of the multidisciplinary PHCT. Nurses have guidance on this matter from the United Kingdom Central Council for Nursing, Midwifery and Health Visiting (UKCC), as set out in Clause 10 of the *Code of professional conduct*,[35] which makes it quite clear that confidentiality can be breached only in extraordinary circumstances.

In 1993, a document, *Confidentiality and people under 16*, was circulated to all GPs and FHSAs.[36] The document gives clear guidance to GPs about young people, regardless of age, consenting to treatment; about their right to confidentiality and their right to consult another GP for contraceptive services. Young people often find it difficult to seek contraceptive advice from their general practice. This may be because they find the practice unwelcoming and difficult to access. Additionally, many young people still have the mistaken fear that their GP and the practice team will not respect their confidentiality. Rumours are spread among groups of young people:

'I went to see my doctor, and the receptionist asked me if my mum knew that I was here.'

'I can't go and see my GP, he is very friendly with my parents and would tell them.'

If young people are going to come to the practice for contraceptive advice, it is essential that they are made to feel welcome and understand that anything they say will be treated in total confidence.

Older people may fear that information will be disclosed to their partner or other family member – or they may feel the subject is too personal to discuss with someone they know.

Legal issues and accountability

The UKCC regulates the actions of nurses and produces a number of documents which offer guidance. The most relevant here are:

*   *Guidelines for professional practice*[37]

*   *Code of professional conduct* (1996)[35]

*   *Standards for the administration of medicines*[38]

*   *Standards for records and record keeping.*[39]

A further document, entitled *Exercising accountability,*[40] sets out a framework for considering ethical aspects of professional practice.

The *Code of professional conduct*[35] is the definitive document with regard to how a nurse is expected to conduct herself during the course of her work. It provides the basis on which any misconduct will be judged. It clearly states that each nurse is personally accountable for her own actions and it would not be accepted for her to claim that she behaved in a particular way because she was told to by a doctor or any other person. This includes acknowledging any limitations to her own knowledge or competence and as such she should not undertake any activity that she is not trained for and competent to carry out.

This clearly covers the situation where a nurse in general practice is performing tasks or duties that she is not trained to do and would include carrying out 'pill checks' or giving telephone advice on contraception with no training.

5

The role of other key members of the primary health care team

Practice manager

The development of the practice manager's role over the last 5–10 years has been rapid, and standards of candidates presenting at interview seem to get higher and higher. It is not unusual, particularly in large practices, to meet practice managers holding a string of professional business qualifications, including an MBA. Their role in the business planning and marketing aspects of the service is likely to be invaluable. For an up-to-date view of the practice manager's role the reader is referred to Drury and Hobden-Clarke's *The practice manager.*[41]

The practice manager's wholehearted cooperation is vital; he or she should be closely involved in organizing the family planning service and should play a key part in any discussions about how the service might be improved. The practice manager is responsible for ensuring that the system of recording claims is accurate, whether manual or computerized (see Chapter 7). He or she must carry out a reconciliation every quarter to ensure that all claims made have been paid. All these tasks may be delegated, depending on the size and manpower resource of the practice, but the practice manager should be responsible for the overall control of these support systems.

Health visitor

Health visitors have a great deal of contact with fertile women through monitoring of child development. They have a crucial role in the initiation and continuation of use of contraception after childbirth. They often pick up family and marital problems, including sexual difficulties. They provide helpful liaison in relation to women who undergo repeated unintended pregnancy. Because of their close contact with mothers who are breast-feeding, they must keep up to date with contraception during lactation. Much of their continuing education is in connection with child development, child protection and so on.

There are many opportunities for involving health visitors in the development of the family planning service. The types of planning discussion outlined in Chapter 8 may be extended to include the health visitor. It may also be appropriate for the GP and/or practice nurse playing the lead role in family planning to conduct some in-house training for health visitors and other members of the PHCT.

Midwife

The midwife's contact with women is episodic and their role in the post-partum period is minimal as they withdraw at 10 days post-partum. However, they play a useful part in focusing a woman's thoughts on the method she wishes to use after delivery. Some un-intended pregnancies result from a hiatus in care between delivery and the postnatal check up (if attended). A plan can be made during pregnancy and can be carried through by whichever member of the PHCT seems appropriate.

Discussion of contraception can usefully be included in the practice's maternity protocol for, say, the 30-week antenatal visit. (There is nothing in the regulations to say that a fee claim cannot be made when a patient is pregnant.)

Regarding both health visitor and midwife, important policy matters may be specified in the contracts with the community trust for standard and community fundholders.

School nurse

The school nurse is the only person working within the school setting who can offer specific confidential medical advice to individual pupils. This is a vital service as pupils will often not feel able to raise personal worries in a classroom session. (Teachers and other health professionals working in schools can only give general information to pupils about contraception and where confidential advice may be obtained.)

Many schools now provide drop-in health sessions, run by the school nurse where young people can seek advice and information on any health issue. These sessions give young people the opportunity to obtain confidential sexual health advice from the nurse without anyone knowing why they are attending.

The school nurse will usually have the trust of teachers in most of the schools she covers. She can play a vital role by supporting the work of teachers; she can act as a resource for them and also deliver some of the sex education for them. However she is constrained by what content the school governors decide is permissible beyond the National Curriculum.

School nurses can foster links between the school and local PHCTs. Local sexual health services report a rise in teenagers seeking advice where these links are made.

Receptionist

An account of the changing role of the receptionist in general practice over the last 5 years is given in the *Medical receptionists and secretaries handbook*.[42]

Patients judge a practice by their first impressions and its external appearance. The practice should ensure that all patients are dealt with promptly, efficiently and courteously.

Receptionists wield considerable power as they can ration appointments and create a barrier to access. They have a difficult job balancing the pressure from patients to be seen quickly and the inevitably finite number of urgent appointments available on a particular day. They need specific training in how to judge which requests are urgent and in telephone skills. This is particularly important in relation to emergency contraception.

An innovation here is the emergency contraception card (Figure 5.1). This confidentiality card can overcome one of the major obstacles to accessing the service – embarrassment. The card can be made available inside a leaflet explaining the availability of emergency contraception. Production of the card at the reception area leads to access to an on-the-day appointment. Provision can be made on the card for the woman to fill in her name and address, making any interrogation at the desk unnecessary. It is hoped that these cards will help to improve access to services, especially in the vulnerable under-16 age group.

The Black Country Family Practice

Confidentiality Card

If you require emergency contraception and you feel too embarrassed to tell the receptionist, just hand over this card and we will ensure you are seen by a doctor that day.

If you want to, you can write your name and address on the back of the card rather than having to say it out loud to the receptionist.

Let's talk about sex!

Services

- Counselling
- Contraception
- Advice
- Sexual health checks
- Preconception counselling

Emergency contraception:

This is a method of contraception which can be taken following sex and works if taken within 3 days to prevent an unwanted pregnancy.

Under certain circumstances a coil can be fitted up to 5 days after unprotected sex to prevent an unwanted pregnancy.

Remember

Every consultation with your doctor is private and we will not tell anyone else about it without your permission.

☆ **THIS ALSO APPLIES IF YOU ARE UNDER 16.** ☆

Figure 5.1: The confidential emergency contraception card is contained in this four-page leaflet. Courtesy of Dr Tony Robinson.

Receptionists need to understand the different lengths of appointment set for different procedures and routine follow-up intervals. They should know the practice policy on issuing contraceptive pills when a woman rings up having completely finished her supplies. See also details on setting up telephone helplines in the case of pill, and related, scares (Chapter 2) – the receptionist will need to be part of the team following the agreed protocol.

6

Family planning outside the practice setting

Family planning clinics

Trust clinic services are changing. There is now a career structure for medical staff. The Faculty of Family Planning and Reproductive Health Care of the RCOG was founded in March 1993. A membership examination – membership of the Faculty of Family Planning (MFFP) – has been established and a higher specialist training programme has been drawn up. All that remains is to fit this into the Calman system of training and the Specialist Register.

Consultants in family planning/reproductive health care/sexual health or community gynaecology are the fastest growing group of consultants in UK medicine. There are thought to be 67 existing posts (as at February 1997) and community trusts are giving these posts a high priority. The standard of specialist services should rise. Such services will hopefully include a psychosexual problem clinic; some will offer sterilization. These consultants are a source of advice with problem cases and often referral to them will be more appropriate than to the gynaecology service.

There is a need for more support for the PHCT from trust services with telephone advice, training, updating and publicity for contraceptive services. It is vital that the PHCT and trust family planning services work together to provide a service to the local community.

Gynaecologists

In some areas, acute unit specialists may still be doing colposcopy, abortions and infertility care, but in future this work will tend to take place under the auspices of the community units. Sterilization may differ from area to area, depending on the surgical experience of the family planning consultant. Some gynaecology departments run an emergency contraception service.

Accident and emergency departments

Some A&E departments provide emergency contraception; some are resolutely against the concept. Commissioning authorities should ask A&E departments to formulate a policy that fits in with provision by other local providers. Keep up to date with local hospital policies as these often change as doctors rotate.

Genitourinary medicine

There is a great deal of overlap between GUM and family planning. A recent trend has been the merger of, or intensive cooperation between, genitourinary medicine and family planning services. Such joint services may be under the same roof or in separate premises but close together. Such combined services now operate in a number of areas in the UK.

A characteristic of a genitourinary service is its centralization. Adequate laboratory backup on site is essential, and specially trained health workers are required to carry out contact tracing. Unlike family planning – which can be provided in local areas or on a domiciliary basis – genitourinary work has to be central.

Many patients will discuss their risk of exposure to sexually transmitted infection (STI) in the context of contraception. It is important that the PHCT understands its limitations with regard to diagnosis and treatment of STIs and has a low threshold for referral to GUM.

Young persons' centres

Practices may want to liaise with the staff of youth centres or clubs in connection with family planning and related educational activities or information on local services. Young persons' centres are often only open for limited times.

Schools

GPs may be called upon to give talks to pupils or to educate teachers. Such invitations are a splendid opportunity to ensure that up-to-date information reaches school children. But sex education is a lot more than facts. It is vital that classes work on negotiating skills and attitudes to sexuality and this will require sustained teaching, usually by the personal and social education teacher.

Health promotion unit

The health promotion section of every health authority is the source of the CES leaflets which are so invaluable in family planning (see p. 25). Encourage the practice secretarial staff to develop a good rapport with the health promotion staff! Material about national advertising campaigns can be supplied and make a striking display on the surgery noticeboards.

Health authority

Family health services authorities in England and Wales have now merged with district health authorities to form unified health authorities. As well as providing our pay they have much to offer in terms of resources in the development of practices and locally-based staff training.

Charitable organizations

Non-profit-making charities such as the British Pregnancy Advisory Service and Marie Stopes offer a wide range of services, including pregnancy testing, sterilization, sterilization reversal and abortion (see Useful addresses, p. 119). There are branches in major towns and cities throughout the UK. Historically, the charities have filled a gap in the NHS services and sadly, in some parts of the country, they continue to do so. Some patients opt to bypass their GP, pay for the services and achieve complete anonymity.

Some health authorities contract with charities for abortion services. Charities often have specialized centres that carry out second-trimester abortions. Fundholding practices may use their budget for purchasing abortions in this sector.

Brook Advisory Centres

Brook is the only network of centres in this country offering young people free and confidential contraceptive and counselling services. Eighteen branches in the UK manage 36 centres, funded locally by health authorities. Nationally, Brook runs a helpline with a series of recorded messages on sexual health topics. This is publicized weekly to the readers of the teenage magazines *Just* 17 and *More*. Over 34 000 calls are registered each year.

Pharmacists

There are over 12 000 community pharmacies in Britain, visited by 6 million people every day. Pharmacists are sometimes considered as part of the PHCT but this happens only in some very enlightened practices.

Pharmacies are a powerful outlet for educational material. The FPA regularly produces such material for the Pharmacy Healthcare Scheme. In November 1994 around 600 000 leaflets on emergency contraception were distributed through this scheme.

Some 55% of pharmacists are reported to get regular requests for information on emergency contraception. Pharmacists also advise on home pregnancy tests that they sell or will perform pregnancy tests themselves. They sell many over-the-counter (OTC) contraceptive products, as mentioned in Chapter 3. They also have computerized records of all prescriptions dispensed and can check for drug interactions for those receiving hormonal contraception.

Under the Medicines Act 1968, retail pharmacists can supply a prescription-only medicine as an emergency supply made at the request of a patient.[43] The conditions that apply to this procedure are:

- the patient's GP must be registered in the UK

- the pharmacist ascertains there is immediate need for the medicine

- the product has been previously prescribed for the patient.

For most drugs the maximum quantity that can be dispensed is five days' supply, but the oral contraceptive is an exception to this rule and a full cycle can be given. This facility is perhaps not widely known to the public. Greater dissemination of this information might help the problem of missed pills when women are travelling in the UK away from home.

Replacement diaphragms and caps can also be sold, provided the size is known by the patient.

7

Information technology

Faxes

Fax and computers have changed the face of society and no less so in medicine. A fax is often a better medium than the telephone for urgent appointments and can be transmitted into 'safe havens' where there is no risk of the contents being seen by any unauthorized person. Incoming faxes are now the official route for the 'cascade' which flows top down from the Department of Health via Directors of Public Health in the event of urgent notifications such as 'pill scares', as mentioned in Chapter 2. In October 1995 this cascade operated in a patchy fashion, but in June 1996, for the first time, it all ran smoothly.

Trends in general practice computing

Ninety-two per cent of practices are set to have computers by 1997. The decision these days is not whether to computerize but how far to computerize. The degree of computerization is very much a personal matter; there will be less gain, for example, for single-handed practices.[44] Full computerization must have the support of the whole PHCT. The applications of computers mentioned in this chapter are based upon a high level of commitment.

With around 50 GP computer systems available today, no specific software can be recommended. Software is ever evolving and as in other fields the Windows environment is taking over from MS-DOS and UNIX (XENIX) operating systems. Software should use Read codes because these have been in use as the NHS official coding system since 1990.

There are approximately half a million Read codes. The family planning codes in the four-character system are at present deficient in some respects, for example, in relation to subdermal implants.

Five-character Read codes, which are gradually replacing the original four-character codes, allow much greater detail in coding. Newer versions of Read codes (version three to be released in March 1997) allow cross-referencing with Office of Population, Censuses and Surveys (OPCS) and International Classification of Diseases (ICD) codes and access via synonyms, for example. Version three is needed if a practice is to become truly paperless. At present there are difficulties with data exchange between practices with different versions of the Read codes.

More and more, practices are replacing a multi-user system comprising dumb terminals with intelligent terminals (workstations) with a graphical user interface system that forms a network. The advantage of having a PC on the desk is that a floppy disk or CD-ROM can be put into a drive and used for the benefit of the patient who is consulting. A program about a particular method or missed pills rules (Figure 7.1)[45] can be run, an electronic textbook referred to or a program showing the anatomy of an appropriate part of the body can be

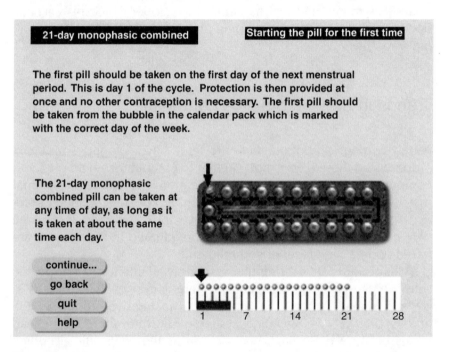

Figure 7.1: The Oral Contraceptive Help Program developed by Medi Cine International for Schering Health Care Ltd assists general practices in providing comprehensive advice both for women starting the pill for the first time and those experiencing problems.

displayed. All the Contraceptive Education Service leaflets are now included in a patient information system called *Patient wise*, available as a floppy disk-based datafile which can be printed out in front of the patient.[46]

A good package will offer software modules that have several functions. Increasing amounts of software are available on CD-ROM and a CD-ROM drive in the PC is becoming essential. The capacity of a single 74-minute compact disc is roughly equivalent to 472 high-density floppy disks or 272 000 pages of text. Files cannot be deleted, are impervious to viruses and have an estimated life of up to 100 years.

The consultation

The package should allow entry of as much free text as the operator wishes. There should be a facility for producing user-defined screens (templates) for clinical protocols such as initiating oral contraception. A practice protocol should be written that clarifies how data entry is to be uniformly carried out so that coding is accurate and meaningful reports can be subsequently run.

The downside is that the computer can interfere significantly with the flow of communication in the consultation and ideally most of the data entry should be carried out after the patient has left the room.

Prescribing

The package should contain a comprehensive hierarchical drug dictionary, based on the *British National Formulary*, for easy prescribing. There should be an alert system so that a drug being prescribed is checked against repeat medication and all drug interactions are flagged. In addition, ideally, the drugs prescribed should also be checked against the patient's medical history so that contraindications are flagged too.

The package should have a repeat prescribing facility, although this does not play a major part in family planning. As the products are cheap compared with other drugs it makes sense to prescribe quantities sufficient for the interval between visits. Normally pill repeats are for 24 or 28 weeks. This is because patients should come in for a blood pressure check every 6 months.

Practice administration

At registration a woman's method of contraception can be coded and entered on the database, taking the information from new patient registration questionnaires. The registration facility in the system should also include a category for patients registered for general medical services at other practices who choose to come to your practice for contraceptive services. Within the practice computer system there should be a diary function for automatic recall of patients due for checks and for item-of-service fee expiry. An appointments system that can be accessed from all terminals is also useful.

A word processor is necessary for generating predefined letters. A report generator is needed for running electronic audits, checking claims, producing needs assessment data and other functions, such as identifying those on a particular brand of pill in the event of a scare.

The system should allow aggregated patient data to be merged into spreadsheet and word processing packages. Lastly, desk-top publishing allows superb quality newsletters or posters to be designed – important assets in the promotion of the family planning service.

Training

Computer programs, such as Organon's 'DFFP case studies', are extremely valuable material for initial training or updating and are just as useful for nurses as for doctors.[47] Distance learning is a big growth area ideal for multi-media. Family planning is likely to see this soon.

Electronic data interchange

The Links project uses the Racal Healthlink network to 'hook up' the practice to the health authority, with each participant having their own secure 'mailbox'. The practice computer can be linked directly with that of the health authority so that registrations and item-of-service payments can be electronic, saving time and paper, and in the long-term reducing the likelihood of error. Other outside bodies can be similarly accessed, as shown in Figure 7.2. Communications with pathology laboratories allow blood test results to be entered process of business planning has been well documented in a number of primary care texts. The guidance given in *Business and health planning for general practice*[49] is especially helpful, particularly the formats and checklists given in the appendices. The fundamental basis of all practice plans is a straightforward, logical approach:

- Where are we now?
- Where do we want to be?
- How can we get there?
- Which way is best?
- How can we ensure arrival?

Note that one of the strongest 'drivers' in general practice is the enthusiasm and interests of individual GPs and practice staff, since it is this that governs the evolution of not just one service or another but of the practice as a whole. Formal business planning, following this five-pronged approach, should not stifle this enthusiasm, interest and creativity. Rather, it should enable the practice to review its assets, strengths and weaknesses in an objective way, and then move forward by capitalizing on those assets in the most effective (or strategic) way and by focusing on long-term goals – both personal and practice ones – as well as immediate needs.

It must be recognized that good communication is a fundamental part of the planning process since, if the business plan is communicated to all the practice staff, it can give everybody a sense of shared purpose, a common goal and the basis for team-working. You should therefore concentrate upon developing the plan not in isolation but by involving all the practice staff.

Today it is mandatory for all fundholding practices to provide a formal business plan but this is not true of non-fundholding practices, who are required only to complete an Annual Report, pre-structured by the health authority.

Where are we now?

The starting point of the planning process is a SWOT analysis, which is designed to provide you with a detailed insight into the practice's

---

The Internet	Databases such as MedLine
Trusts	Primary health care team
Health authority	Pathology laboratories

Figure 7.2: Information technology enables the practice to process data quickly and efficiently with a range of organizations and services.

directly into patients' individual files, obviating the need for data entry from a paper record. Databases can be searched for information to enable evidence-based medicine to be practised. NHS trusts can be accessed too.

NHSnet is a secure national network developed exclusively for the NHS. This type of network is also referred to as an Intranet – this provides a similar range of communication and information services to a closed group as the Internet does for the general public. An Intranet uses the same sort of software tools but operates within a secure and controlled environment. Within this structure, medical records can be transferred from practice to practice. Appointment booking can be changed from fax to electronic exchange.

Connection to *NHSnet* will support access to national, regional and local applications and local area network connections. There will be considerable savings in time and resources. Access will only be provided for NHS organizations or others meeting a code of connection. Through *NHSnet* it will be possible to access *NHSweb* which is to include knowledge bases, bulletin boards, education and training material and electronic books.

Electronic data interchange raises confidentiality issues. Patients must be assured that their consultations are totally confidential. We must be convinced that systems are secure before adopting them. To this end the Faculty of Family Planning and Reproductive Health Care has set up an Information Management and Technology Working Group to look at the implications of computerization.

The Internet is a worldwide communications network linking together millions of computers via telephone lines. It consists of a number of facilities such as E-mail, file transfer facilities and the World Wide Web. These facilities allow information to be sent, received and viewed almost instantaneously anywhere in the world. The Internet's component networks are individually run by governments, academic, commercial and voluntary organizations. Individuals can link to this matrix of networks by using their PC, a modem and an Internet connection provided by an Internet service provider. Recent surveys suggest that there are currently over 20 million people with access to the Internet and over 30 million E-mail addresses worldwide. The number of connections is doubling every few months and it is predicted that there will be over 200 million people connected by 2002.

All users who are linked to the Internet are provided with an E-mail address or postbox. Sending messages and computer files by E-mail costs only the price of a local telephone call and is thus far cheaper than post or longer-distance telephone calls.

Internet sites have already been established by the World Health Organization, the Department of Health, the *British Medical Journal*, and the *Lancet*. The National Coordinating Unit for Clinical Audit in Family Planning in Hull has already made audit contacts via the Internet.

It is likely that, in future, the Department of Health will send out urgent messages through E-mail. This will be much quicker than faxing and will cut out the health authority stage; the same message can be sent out to all practices and relevant trust clinics simultaneously. The proviso is that all practices are computerized and linked to the Internet; the author predicts that this will become a condition of running a practice by the turn of the century.

Instead of sending for journal articles, leaflets and booklets, they can be retrieved from the Internet instantaneously. Sites called up on the Internet will, in the future, be an integral part of patient learning, replacing books and CD-ROMs.

The range of health information services available to the general public is huge and the quality varies from excellent to awful. There is not, and probably never will be, any form of regulation, and this is a concern to many health professionals. At the time of writing one of the most comprehensive guides to information on women's health issues, including contraception, on the Internet is in *Your personal net doctor*.[48] This 350-page paperback has been edited by a US doctor, and includes dozens of international sites of use to both doctors and patients. Whilst some of this information 'travels', US information may contradict UK practice.

New sites are set up in their dozens every week, and current sites are being constantly upgraded and improved. It is possible to spend hours gazing into the screen!

8

Planning for patient-centred care

Maggie Pettifer

Although many GPs claim to be patient-centred in their approach to family planning, in reality there is often scope for improvement. Perhaps the family planning clinic is at fixed times each week and many patients may want, but are unable to, attend. The difference between GP-centred care and patient-centred care may be illustrated by these two sets of beliefs:

GP-centred care:

'There is no good reason to change because we are the best practice locally.'

'Apart from occasional problems the "system" works really well.'

'Patients can sometimes be a nuisance.'

'As GPs we know what is best for patients.'

Patient-centred care:

'We need to understand clearly patients' spoken, and unspoken, needs and expectations of the service. We are willing to go out of our way to find out what those needs and expectations are.'

'We need to learn from other practices across the country and to integrate in our practice what has worked well elsewhere. We welcome the development of new services.'

'Without our patients there would be no healthcare system and no progress or change.'

This chapter is about evaluating the family planning service you currently offer and then looking at ways in which it can be improved, in line with patient needs and expectations, i.e. patient-centred care. The way in which market research, and specifically the use of questionnaires, contributes to this process is outlined on p. 67. The

strengths and weaknesses, and the external opportunities and threats that confront it. This simple framework is used widely throughout businesses, charities and the public sector.

Simple though it is, the SWOT analysis has often been abused and misused, with results so bland and meaningless that they are not worth taking any further. The following points will help to ensure that your practice SWOT provides the basis for a workable action plan.

1   Never conduct the SWOT analysis on your own; always do so in group discussion with your PHCT. All views and insights must be considered. Always review your SWOT factors on an annual, or more frequent, basis.

2   Always look at the strengths and weaknesses from the viewpoint of the patient. In this way you can avoid making a series of bland, reassuring statements about the service, and rather concentrate upon how it is really seen from the outside in.

3   Start with a broadly unstructured approach in order to get the ideas flowing, but gradually pull the points together under a series of headings such as:

    –   the quality of doctor–patient interaction

    –   the quality of nurse–patient interaction

    –   the support and administration systems and procedures

    –   how well IT is being used

    –   how well the service is promoted

    –   the service provided by local 'competition'

    –   the part of the 'market' locally you currently do not serve

    –   and so on.

4   Avoid the temptation simply to list strengths, weaknesses, opportunities and threats. A false sense of satisfaction can be gained if the strengths and opportunities outweigh numerically the weaknesses and threats. Far more important is an appreciation of the significance of each SWOT factor. Attaching some kind of priority score to each factor listed is helpful. Certainly it pays to rank them in some order of significance.

5   It also pays to be ruthless and weed out any factors which are interesting but simply irrelevant to the practice for the time being.

6   When considering threats and opportunities, you need to take quite a broad view of factors outside the practice at both a local and national level. Nobody has a crystal ball, but it helps to anticipate likely future changes in the external environment. The types of factors you may consider include: government policy, legislation, the results of clinical trials, guidelines from evidence-based medicine, the national press, available products and products likely to be launched, financial considerations such as reimbursement, the changing needs and attitudes of women.

7   The final step of a SWOT analysis is often missed out. It involves linking each strength to a matching opportunity, deciding how each weakness can be overcome, or minimized, and thinking about how to reduce or neutralize each threat, or even how to turn it into an opportunity. Here is an example showing how a strength in a family planning service, perceived by patients, can be coupled to an opportunity:

Strength: The family planning service is offered in a convenient location, familiar to patients; practice staff are known to patients as are the procedures.

Opportunity: The local college has just got university status and is set to double in size in the next five years.

Implication: Capitalize on existing strengths to extend the family planning service to a new incoming population.

The following SWOT factors have been collected from a wide range of practices, and are listed to give you an idea of what to look for. Bear in mind that they may not apply to your practice at all, and many factors not listed may be absolutely crucial in your planning process.

Examples of strengths – always match these to opportunities

•   The family planning service is offered in a convenient location, familiar to patients; practice staff are known to patients, as are the procedures.

•   The patients who use the service believe the advice they get is up-to-date and to be trusted; they can rely on what the GP or nurse tells them about current opinion as to the safety and efficacy of contraceptives.

- Women know they are offered more choice of contraception in this practice than anywhere else in the vicinity.

Examples of weaknesses – how may these be minimized or overcome?

- The family planning clinic is at fixed times each week and it may be difficult for some women to fit in with clinic times.

- The practice has not addressed the need for improved communication with its ethnic minority groups, or indeed really listened to their views about the type of service and advice they need. Language has also been a problem.

- The staff running the clinics are often asked technical questions by patients which they are unable to answer. A small but growing group of patients seems to know more about recent trials than the GPs!

- Two pill scares have happened over the last 18 months and the practice was unprepared. There is no 'crisis management' plan at the ready.

Examples of opportunities – link these to practice strengths

- An increasingly wide range of contraceptive choices is available, which means you can customize the service much more closely to the needs of each woman.

- The local college has just acquired university status and is doubling in size over the next 5 years.

- The new female partner who has just joined the practice is interested in teenage health, and has been involved in writing and research in this area.

- There is a captive market of registered patients and a potential ('unserved') market among the patients of other GPs in the locality who currently appear to offer a less patient-friendly and comprehensive service.

Examples of threats – these need to be overcome, or possibly turned into an opportunity

*   The family planning clinics, having declined in the 1980s, seem to be getting their act back together and may attract customers away from your practice.

*   There are noises about introducing a limited list once again.

*   A pharmaceutical representative for a company that markets an IUD warns that you have not seen the end of the pill scares. Apparently another 'adverse' meta-analysis is likely to be published in 4 months' time.

The use of market research in evaluating the family planning service

One of the conventional wisdoms in marketing is that you can never ask too many questions before you make strategic moves. The best quality information is gained from objective research, mainly in the form of written questionnaires completed by patients (see Appendix 1).

There are two steps in evaluating the family planning service in your practice.

1   You should evaluate the attitudes of patients *who already use* the service in order to arrive at a measure of user satisfaction. Some may attend a dedicated clinic and some may use the drop-in approach. You can reach all the patients who use the service by mail (it is courteous – and improves the response rate – to include an s.a.e. for return of the form, or, better still, a Freepost address). Alternatively you can reach all those who visit within, say, a 6-week period by adding an explanation during the consultation of why you need their input on a questionnaire, ensuring that they receive the questionnaire before leaving the surgery. If the questionnaire is short and simple they may be asked to complete it there and then. It is essential to state that information gathered from any of these survey methods is confidential.

2   You should evaluate the views of all those patients *who could use* the service within the practice population but who currently do not, using your computer database to identify them. Great care

must be taken to ensure that women are not approached who, for example, cannot conceive, have had a hysterectomy, or similar. Considerable thought must also be given to the question of how, if at all, you approach young women living with their parents. The only way to access all potential users of the service is by mail. This may seem expensive, but this must be balanced against the increase in practice revenue gained by attracting more users to the service. One way you can test the value of a mailed questionnaire is to select a pilot group comprising, say, 20% of the final group, and mail this subgroup first.

Market research is a fascinating and complex skill. Its value in general practice is described in *Marketing and general practice*.[50] Many of the concepts in this book are described in greater depth in *Strategic marketing management*.[51]

We are all aware of the way consumers are deluged with questionnaires, and patients are no exception. It helps if the questionnaire is thoughtfully designed, produced imaginatively on a desk-top publishing package, and sent out with a clear, informative letter. You might want to indicate the time frame for rolling out the new service, or provide some information about good aspects ('strengths') of the existing service. It helps to tell patients either verbally or in writing why their views are indispensable in improving the service.

As well as formal questionnaires, it is also useful to glean market intelligence information, particularly about threats and opportunities. You can find out a lot about what else is happening locally from colleagues and from your health authority. Pharmaceutical company representatives visit all the practices in their territory and therefore have a good 'bird's eye view' of service delivery, new facilities, innovative ideas, and so on. Keep up to date by reading journals and newsletters and by networking.

Lastly, it is possible to convene focus groups of patients to facilitate the process of patient-led care. The problem here is that patients who have been in the practice for years simply may not have the insight to know 'how good, good may be', or what exists elsewhere that is better. The set-up time and management of focus groups are quite onerous, and reporting on the results is time-consuming, so focus groups for a single practice are probably unrealistic. However, every 2 years or so, it may be well worth setting up a combined focus group as part of locality commissioning, or accessing information from focus groups set up by the health authority to support locality commissioning.

There is some evidence that moving patients out of the care setting, and away from their professional advisers, to a focus group run by a third party provides the most accurate picture of what patients think about the service provided, and particularly about the manner and mannerisms of the staff they encounter. If you are prepared to act on the feedback such a group provides, and with colleagues fund the expense, then it could be useful.[52] This links in with research studies – see p. 82.

Planning the future of the service

When you have conducted your SWOT analysis, ranked your SWOT factors in importance, linked strengths to opportunities, taken a view on how to minimize threats or turn them to your advantage, and how to overcome weaknesses, it is time to move forward and plan to improve service, in terms of size, scope, quality, flexibility, or all of these.

Where do we want to go?

The next stage is to set some clear objectives. They should probably fill no more than two sheets of paper. The following pointers may be helpful:

1   Start with the most crucial objective and work down to the least critical one.

2   State each objective very specifically in such a way that progress can be measured. Many plans talk in relative terms such as 'better', 'optimize', 'more', and so on. The plan should define where you are right now (point A) and where you want to get to (point B) in very specific terms. This may sound pedantic, but only by writing plans in this way can you judge if you have made any progress.

3   Keep the number of objectives down – no more than 12.

4   Ensure each one is workable in terms of the practice's strengths and assets, the environmental opportunities, NHS legislation, and any other constraints. It would be foolish to follow all the

ideas covered in this book and then come up with a plan that was light years removed from the existing assets of your practice.

5   Ensure objectives are compatible with each other.

6   Each objective should fit within the time frame of your plan – if you review progress annually then each objective should be achievable in that time.

7   The list of objectives for the family planning service should fit with the business plan for the practice as a whole. You cannot expand and improve every service in the practice at the same time. It might be best to work up gradually to your ideal family planning service over, say, a period of 3 years, if other services are to be upgraded even more urgently.

8   The list of objectives should be developed in consultation with the practice team.

When the list of objectives is complete you are in a position to review whether or not it is entirely realistic, either in terms of magnitude or in terms of time frame. In doing this you are trying to identify the nature and significance of any gaps that exist between what is currently available in the practice (staff, IT, equipment, cash, premises) and what is needed. The resource implications of your plan may be zero – the objectives relate simply to doing things a different, and better, way. Alternatively the resource implications may be substantial. In this case you have to decide whether to water down your objectives, argue the case more strongly with colleagues (who may not be in favour of your plan), or lengthen the timescale. The benefit of setting objectives, and weighing up the resource implications, is that you foresee problems before making substantial changes, and particularly before incurring major expense.

How are we going to get there?

Having identified your objectives you should be in a position to develop a written action plan. For each objective state the actions needed to achieve the objective, who is responsible for each action, and what measures of performance are necessary. Implementation is the hardest part of the planning process as you move away from all the rigours of analysis and the excitement of a vision for the future to actually doing it.

It helps to have brief review meetings, and constantly refer back to the short, simple, clear objectives, to acknowledge where real progress has been made. How do you know if real progress has been made?

Measuring progress

If the objectives for improving the family planning service have been written in very specific terms, then it will be easy to compare the past with the present, and see if progress has been made. The tools to measure progress are:

- practice records – financial and statistical

- patient feedback – anecdotal and formally researched

- staff feedback – anecdotal and formally researched

- a log of unexpected problems encountered in the roll-out of the service

- increase or decrease in the uptake of the service

- perceived image of the practice as a whole

- retaliatory action by other local service providers.

Promoting your improved family planning service

Once the practice has upgraded its family planning service this is the time to communicate the improvements, and more importantly the benefits of the improvements, to the customer.

The facilities, the staff, the training, the systems, should be in place before you promote the service. As a customer it is very irritating to encounter teething problems and badly thought out concepts and system, even as you sit reading a brochure extolling the benefits of the 'new system'!

Ways in which the improved family planning service can be promoted include:

- positive messages from practice staff when talking about the service, always concentrating on the benefits of the service, and its capacity/scope to offer a better service to both existing, and new, patients

- posters

- brochures on specific services

- entry in the practice brochure and newsletter

- entry in a guide to your area, such as a local town/city map

- entry in a local newspaper

- telling the Family Planning Association

- inclusion in information provided by Regional Health Care Helplines

- entry in local directories, e.g. local student directories.

Planning pays off

Progress is never 100% as you planned, and every review of progress reveals more strengths, weaknesses, opportunities and threats than you had imagined. Reviews give you the opportunity to acknowledge the real progress that has been made and, importantly, the contribution of staff in reaching these goals. They also give you the chance to refocus the strategy for the next 2 years. Improvement is a lifelong process. The competitive pressures between practices and services will intensify in the years to come. The discipline of planning, with particular attention to patients' needs and expectations, is a sound basis for success.

9

Quality issues

Clinical effectiveness

Clinical effectiveness comprises two main parts: knowing what one should be doing (doing the right thing) and being able to implement that knowledge (doing the thing right). The first consists of commissioning research, publicizing the results and translating them into clinical guidelines. The second consists of diffusing and disseminating this knowledge so that it is incorporated into everyday practice; this practice is then evaluated using clinical audit and by monitoring performance, and finally outcome is measured (Figure 9.1).

Improving clinical effectiveness is currently being given a high profile and priority by the NHS Executive. A coordinated approach is being used which brings together research evidence, clinical guidelines, clinical audit and outcome assessment to ensure that patients have access to health care of proven quality and the greatest benefit can be realized from available resources. Support is being given to R&D programmes which are dedicated to the production of clinical guidelines and clinical audit and the development of outcome measures.

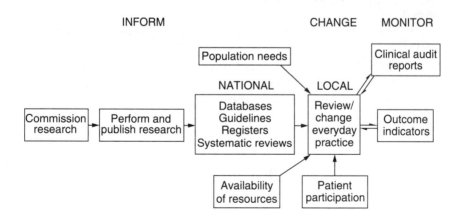

Figure 9.1: The process of achieving clinical effectiveness.

Protocols (local guidelines)

The importance of protocols to support the family planning service in an individual practice has already been stressed in Chapter 3. The purpose of protocols is to promote effective health care by reinforcing good clinical practice, and to promote change in professionals' practice where this does not comply with recommendations.[53]

Protocols have been shown to contribute to improvement in the quality of care. They may be adapted from national or regional protocols that have been based on literature searches and developed by a multidisciplinary guideline development group, or may be developed *de novo*. Usually there is little point reinventing the wheel, and national or regional protocols can be adapted to acknowledge local or team factors. In the absence of national or regional protocols, local protocols can be developed. An example is shown in Appendix 2.

Protocols should not be introduced without formal discussion with all relevant members of the primary health care team. Protocols should be disseminated (shared and discussed) in order to influence the attitudes, knowledge and understanding of all players in the team.

Implementation programmes are intended to encourage health professionals to change their own clinical practice in line with the protocol. Ownership is the key to effective implementation. Methods of implementation include training, if a new skill is required, adequate organization in the practice to facilitate the change; and possibly computer prompts to remind team members what process has been agreed.

Clinical audit should be used in the implementation of protocols; feedback to individual team members can encourage improved compliance. It also provides team management with the information needed to evaluate the adoption of a protocol and to plan any further steps that may be required to improve performance.

Evidence-based medicine

Some of the activities undertaken in general practice are not based on evidence as there are no randomized clinical trials or epidemiological studies on which to base clinical practice. This cannot be said for family planning. Although not all aspects of family planning are well-researched, the number of papers in the literature is vast. The combined pill is the most researched drug of all. Another point to make here is that not all activities are susceptible to randomized controlled trials and so there will never be this type of evidence available for many aspects of family planning. The Cochrane Database of Systematic Reviews aims to provide the type of information that is needed by clinicians to make decisions about patient care. It is an electronic journal, updated quarterly, of systematic reviews produced by the Cochrane Collaboration – an international network of individuals and institutions committed to preparing, maintaining and disseminating systematic reviews of health care. These reviews are prepared by a group of collaborating authors (a Cochrane Review Group), using explicitly defined methods to reduce the effects of bias. Each review is produced on CD-ROM and put on to the Internet. A Cochrane Fertility Regulation Review Group was formed in Amsterdam in June 1996 and a family planning database will soon be available.

When basing one's clinical practice on evidence, it is important to recognize and be able to state the quality of the evidence. The following grades are used in guideline development, in decreasing order of quality:

- randomized controlled trials (grade A)

- other robust experimental or observational studies (grade B)

- more limited evidence – based on expert opinion and endorsed by respected authorities (grade C).

It is salutary to remember that it was a GP, Dr W M Jordan, who first suspected the link between oral contraceptives and venous thromboembolism and wrote a letter to the *Lancet* in 1961. Epidemiological data since have confirmed this suspicion and the link between the oestrogen component of the pill and venous thromboembolism has been established. Since then, many associations of contraceptive methods with clinical conditions have been postulated. Some have subsequently been proved, some disproved and some are still inconclusive. It is important to remember that there are beneficial effects, as well as adverse effects, of methods of contraception.

In 1968, the Royal College of General Practitioners' (RCGP) oral contraception study was started and it is still continuing. Fourteen hundred GPs recruited 23 000 women who were taking oral contraceptives and a similar number of women who had never taken the pill into a long-term cohort study. Many key papers have been published over the years. A relationship between progestogen dose and arterial disease was established, and the markedly increased risk of circulatory disease in smokers who take the pill was clearly demonstrated too.

These and many other papers from around the world have shaped our thinking and our clinical practice. Progestogen-only methods are far less well-researched. Although there are some metabolic studies, we lack the type of epidemiological information which is available for the combined pill. Case-control studies until recently looked entirely at hospital records.

There is very little research into primary care family planning. There is a UK family planning research network coordinated by the University of Exeter with 23 trust clinics and general practices who collect data, but funding is limited and the scale of the research therefore small. However, useful work has been done and published on various IUDs, the IUS, the acceptability of the female condom, and condom mishaps. Norplant use is also now being studied.

Access to database searches such as MedLine is available through local medical libraries. British Medical Association (BMA) members can link up on-line via a modem to MedLine free of charge. Most of us, however, need assistance from experts to interpret the literature. The Clinical and Scientific Committee of the Faculty of Family Planning has started to put out statements at the time key papers are published. The CSM do so too, as mentioned in the section on the media in Chapter 2. The CSM is the regulatory agency that advises the British Government on drug safety and efficacy and its advice is almost always taken.

The other body that comments on contraceptive products is the European Union's regulatory authority, the Committee for Proprietary Medicinal Products. The CPMP is an arbiter and steps in when national regulatory authorities are not in agreement. After the October 1995 venous thromboembolism scare the CSM issued a statement saying that pills containing gestodene and desogestrel were not to be used by women who had risk factors for venous thromboembolism and should only be used by those who were intolerant of other combined pills and who were prepared to accept an increased risk of thromboembolism. The German equivalent of the CSM issued a similar statement. Regulatory agencies in all other countries in the world at the time of writing (including the CPMP and the United States Food and Drug Administration) were not convinced that the evidence to change prescribing practice was strong enough and reserved judgement pending further data. British GPs would, however, be foolish to pre-scribe against the advice of the CSM, whose guidance would be quoted in English courts.

A great effort has recently been made in relation to prescribing the pill according to evidence[54] rather than anecdote handed down over the years. The conclusions from a consensus conference were:

- taking a personal and family history with particular reference to cardiovascular risk factors and taking an accurate blood pressure measurement are the only two prerequisites for safe provision of the combined pill

- there is no scientific evidence to support any of the following in the routine care of women on the combined pill:
  - pelvic examination
  - teaching breast self-examination/clinical breast examination/mammography
  - urine testing
  - blood testing of any kind
  - weighing.

This will come as a surprise to many. It is often thought that the more screening one does the better. It is important to understand the many negative effects of screening and that many women are put off by the excessive medicalization of contraceptive provision and may discontinue a method because of this.

Other methods are associated with recommendations of best prac-tice. Chlamydia testing has been advocated prior to IUD insertion. According to a theoretical model, testing of women for chlamydia is cost-effective when the prevalence in the population is 6% or more.[55] However, until a well-designed prospective randomized controlled trial shows that testing (and treatment of those positive) of women prior to IUD insertion leads to a reduction in reported incidence of pelvic inflammatory disease, the practice cannot be justified.

Audit

Research and audit are too often confused. Much audit money has been used improperly for small research projects. The term 'medical audit' has been superseded by clinical audit to emphasize the importance of working in a multidisciplinary fashion.

Three constituents of care can be assessed as follows:

1   **Structure** – buildings, equipment, human resources, the records system: the 'environment'. This type of audit tells us nothing about performance

2   **Process** – what the staff in the practice actually do: practice 'activity'

3   **Outcome** – this reflects the benefits of care to the patients. Although the purest form of audit, it is the most difficult. Final outcome is the ultimate measure. In family planning, a high quality service is indicated by a low unplanned pregnancy rate. A zero unplanned pregnancy rate is not attainable; a high quality service allows informed choice and all methods have a failure rate. Outcome indicators are discussed in Chapter 1. 'Intermediate outcome' is a term used to describe a measurable component of care lying between true process and definitive outcome. Intermediate outcome is easier to measure than final outcome and is assumed to predict it, but this may be debatable. Intermediate outcome can be assessed by checking that monitoring and screening have been carried out or by measuring patient satisfaction either using structured interviews (which are expensive and time-consuming) or by self-administered questionnaires.

The audit cycle is shown in Figure 9.2. Audit projects can begin anywhere in the cycle, but to be effective all the steps must be carried out. From April 1996 health authorities have been responsible for funding clinical audit, and NHS regional offices will monitor their performance in developing clinical audit. The National Audit Office recommends closer working between health authorities, fundholders and trusts so that the costs and benefits of clinical audit contribute to improved patient care and provide assurance about the quality of that care.

The National Coordinating Unit for Clinical Audit in Family Planning at the University of Hull produces a 'starter pack' on the basic principles of clinical audit.[56] An emergency contraception audit kit can be ordered from its office which provides comprehensive documentation on how to audit your emergency contraception service. The NCU has developed audit methodology to monitor the reaction to urgent statements from the CSM and other important bodies.

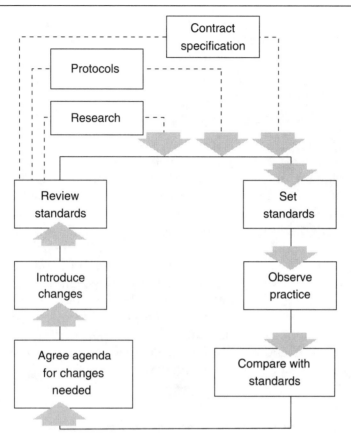

Figure 9.2: Clinical audit cycle. Reproduced with kind permission of the NHS Executive.[57]

Examples of family planning audit which can be carried out in general practice are:

- level 3 PACT data can be examined to check that the practice is not using progestogen-dominant pill brands or that 50 mcg pills are only being used in specific, appropriate cases

- contraceptive advice given at postnatal checks

- knowledge of pill-taking rules

- questionnaire to women who use the family planning service to find out why they use a particular service; also to ascertain whether they think they are receiving a quality service and how it could be improved

- examination of notes of those receiving the combined pill looking at monitoring of smoking status, family history, rubella immune status and blood pressure.

Setting standards

Setting standards locally may well be a practical way to monitor family planning services in general practice and to provide information to users. Standards should be set by clinicians, not by managers. Some health authorities have negotiated voluntary agreements with GPs to set criteria for payment, such as holding a family planning qualification and fitting a minimum number of IUDs each year.

'Sexual health awards' for practices have been developed in one area. These could be extended to include family planning services. A standard and a gold level might be set. The gold level could include regular updating, a trained practice nurse available, at least five IUDs fitted by each doctor undertaking this work per year, sexual health training for GPs and practice nurses and practice policies in place for teenagers and for access to emergency contraception.[58]

Training of general practitioners

Up to 1976 the FPA was the source of training and certificates in family planning. Theoretical training was followed by practical training in family planning clinics on a one-to-one basis with an instructing doctor.

With the formation of the Joint Committee on Contraception of the RCOG, RCGP and FPA, training continued in the same format under this umbrella. With the foundation of the Faculty of Family Planning and Reproductive Health Care of the RCOG in 1993, the certificate of family planning became a diploma (DFFP). The diploma is slightly different in that it is recertifiable every five years.

The RCGP has been concerned with what it terms 'diplomatosis' and maintains that family planning is part of the core content of general practice, and attainment of the MRCGP and the Joint Committee for Postgraduate Training in General Practice (JCPTGP) certificate is evidence of competence to carry out family planning. The responsibility for providing registrars in general practice with theoretical courses lies with the director of postgraduate general practice education, and for practical training with their GP trainer. Nevertheless, diplomatosis is very popular with principals and registrars as evidenced by the 8006 diplomas issued (1997 figure); the majority of these were awarded to doctors working in general practice. Some GPs have become MFFPs too.

Other qualifications awarded by the Faculty are letters of competence in intrauterine techniques and in subdermal contraceptive implant techniques. The Institute of Psychosexual Medicine offers courses of training and issues a certificate of competence to medical practitioners. The DRCOG has family planning in its theoretical syllabus but since 1990 has had no requirement for practical training. There is no formal arrangement for training in operative skills for vasectomy.

A survey of GPs in Wessex found that GPs who held the Joint Committee on Contraception (JCC) certificate offered a wider range of contraceptive services (Table 9.1).

Table 9.1: Percentage of GP holders and non-holders of JCC certificates offering contraceptive services[5]

	JCC holders (%)	Non-holders (%)
Injectables	94	76
Checking IUDs	95	59
Fitting IUDs	82	39
Fitting diaphragms	74	31
Fitting caps	35	15
Sample size	268	130

Training of other members of the PHCT

Training of practice nurses is described in Chapter 4.

Many of the courses helpful to a family planning service are general such as customer care, telephone answering, medical terminology, computer skills, etc. Team-building workshops, with representatives of all types of member attending, can be a particularly powerful way of getting to know each others' roles, developing better channels of communication and working out how to make the practice run more smoothly. In-house training may be very appropriate but protected time must be created.

Teaching

This is likely to be a minority activity for most GPs and nurses, but with the closure of trust clinics some training of doctors and nurses in family planning needs to take place within a general practice setting. GPs can undertake the Faculty's Letter of Competence in Postgraduate Education; and nurses, ENB 997/998: Teaching and Assessing in Clinical Practice. Doctors and nurses in training benefit from seeing the different approach of general practice family planning.

Research

Again this is likely to be a minority activity for most GPs. There is some scope for participating in clinical trials of contraceptive products, but there are strict guidelines and safeguards as well as local ethical approval hurdles.

Anyone considering embarking on such biomedical research should first familiarize themselves with the contents of the World Medical Association Declaration of Helsinki. Consent must be properly informed and subjects must always feel totally free to be released from the study at any time without jeopardizing their care or relationship with their usual medical advisers.

Pharmaceutical companies send clinical research associates to examine the records of those in trials to determine that procedures have been correctly followed and that information is of high quality, with no suspicion that there is any discrepancy between what appears in the clinical notes and the trial proformas.

One of the best introductions to the stages of clinical trials is by Raven in *Clinical trials: an introduction*.[59] Most GPs involved in clinical trials will be involved in phase III trials, usually on quite large patient groups (1000–5000), designed to show the effectiveness, often the relative effectiveness compared with other drugs, and the safety profile. Phase IV trials are conducted after a drug is launched to expand knowledge of drug safety and often to extend the indication range of the product.

Academic research is for the real enthusiast. The main message here is get advice early on in the life of the research project. Help is available from the regional director of postgraduate general practice education, the local university or from one of the larger family planning centres. At a national level, the Faculty of Family Planning and Reproductive Health Care will be able to advise on where help may be obtained.

10

Methods of contraception –
administrative aspects

Since 1975 contraception has been free of charge in general practice, a free service having been introduced into other sectors of the NHS the previous year with the reorganization of the NHS.

Personally administered items

Prescriptions are endorsed by the patient on the back of the FP10 as no-charge contraceptives. Paragraph 44.5 of the *Red Book* (applicable only in England and Wales) states that injections, the IUS, IUDs and contraceptive caps and diaphragms personally administered by a doctor may be claimed for by both dispensing and non-dispensing GPs by using stock kept in the surgery and claiming direct to the Prescription Pricing Authority in Newcastle-upon-Tyne. The prescriptions are sent off with a completed form FP34D.

The basis of reimbursement works in the same way as dispensing:

*   the basic price
*   an on-cost allowance of 10.5% of the basic price
*   a container allowance
*   a dispensing fee
*   an allowance for VAT (payable only to practices not registered for VAT).

So for injectables, the IUS, IUDs, caps and diaphragms, the patient can be saved a trip to a pharmacist and the GP makes a profit.

General practice has been criticized for prescribing a pill-dominated service.[30] Many of the 3 million women on the pill choose to use the GP service and others who want a more specialized service go to a family planning clinic. Whether or not this criticism is founded, effort must be made to provide a comprehensive service offering the whole range of available methods.

The Drug Tariff

Most of us associate the Drug Tariff with a heavy tome of indigestible lists of products distributed every month to all GPs and which over the years must have led to the destruction of many forests!

The Drug Tariff in relation to contraception is a delight to the bureaucrat and a nightmare for doctor and patient. It is totally inappropriate that contraceptive devices are included in this list (they appear between chiropody appliances such as corn plasters and cotton wool!).

All new contraceptive devices have to be approved for use in general practice, although once licensed they are automatically available immediately in both hospitals and clinics. A committee requests evidence of a general demand for the product in general practice. The General Medical Services Committee (GMSC) is consulted, and they like to see letters coming from local medical committees (LMCs) about the particular device. Under this system the Mini-Gravigard device, marketed for a period of 9 years in the UK, was never available to GPs. The longest delays from marketing to Drug Tariff approval were over 8 years for the All-flex arcing spring diaphragm and over 4 years for the copper-T 380 slimline IUD. Luckily, the levonorgestrel intrauterine system (Mirena) was classified as a drug rather than a device because it releases a hormone and so was not subjected to the vagaries of the Drug Tariff.

From June 1998 devices will have to comply with the Medical Devices Regulations and carry the CE mark – a sign that shows the product meets the criteria of the Central European Directive.

Pills

Despite the possibility in 1993 that certain contraceptives were to be added to the selected (limited) list, this action was never taken. All 27 combined pill brands and all six progestogen-only pill brands currently marketed in the UK are prescribable on an FP10.

Injectables

Both injectables available in the UK are prescribable as personally administered items. These are the 12-weekly medroxyprogesterone acetate (Depo-Provera) and the 8-weekly norethisterone oenanthate (Noristerat). However, use of the latter is small in general practice at present. There may be some confusion about what appears in product licences – and hence data sheets/summaries of product characteristics – and what is accepted medical practice.

Both products have been on the market for many years: medroxyprogesterone acetate for over 30 years and norethisterone oenanthate for over 10 years. They are safe drugs and both are recommended in standard family planning texts. It is true that medroxyprogesterone acetate was only licensed as a so-called 'first line' contraceptive in 1995, although it had been licensed for long-term use since 1984. However, it had been prescribed by clinicians (including the author) as a first-line method on a long-term basis in selected cases after counselling before 1984, and norethisterone oenanthate can be prescribed likewise. Reasons for selecting norethisterone oenanthate in preference to medroxyprogesterone acetate include:

• preference for bleeding rather than amenorrhoea

• less chance of spotting

• less risk of marked weight gain

• shorter duration of action if worry about possible side-effects after first injection

• more rapid return of fertility after last injection.

In conclusion, patients who express an interest in injectables as a method should be told of the choice of the two types. Those opting for norethisterone oenanthate should be told about its limited licence (for two injections only) before the injection is given and a note to this effect made in the records.

Subdermal implants

At present only one implant is available. Norplant was launched in the UK in 1993. It cannot be overemphasized that specialized training of health professionals is essential for the success of this method. In a group practice, no more than two GPs should conduct insertions and removals, so that they can retain their skills

At the time of writing about 52 000 implants have been fitted. The launch of Norplant by Hoechst Marion Roussel was a splendid example of excellence in examining and learning from the experience of launches in other countries and then designing an ever expanding 'pyramid' of medical trainers, using theoretical courses and practical training with a model arm. Over 4000 doctors (and a very few nurses) have so far been trained in insertion, but far fewer in removal. About half of all large practices have at least one doctor who is trained in insertion. First-year continuation rates are 85% which is high compared with other methods of contraception. Removal without delay must be offered as an integral part of the service – women must in no way be coerced into continuing.

Health Departments have not agreed any fee for the fitting or removal procedure at the time of writing. This has led to antagonism with the profession as the procedures are time consuming. It is regrettable that the GMSC decreed in September 1995 that GPs should boycott Norplant until a fee structure had been negotiated. They claim that a high fee is warranted because of the risk of possible litigation. Although one firm of solicitors has proposed a class action (collecting together several women who have complained about insertion and removal problems), no class action writs have been issued. In this regard it is interesting to note that in the United States judges in San Francisco, New Jersey and Chicago have all rejected applications for class actions against the US distributor and have ruled that plaintiffs must file individual claims.

Health Departments say that there is no new money for an item-of-service fee. In the meantime, while this stalemate continues, it is British women who suffer by being deprived of a safe and novel form of contraception.

Although there is a high initial cost for this method, when a proper cost–benefit analysis is carried out, including the costs of consultations, dispensing fees and failure of the method, the cost of the subdermal implant is little different from the other hormonal methods.

Intrauterine devices

According to DOH figures, the quality of which is questionable, the number of IUD insertions by GPs in England and Wales rose to a peak of over 500 000 a year in the mid-1980s and then fell to just under 150 000 a year in 1995. This may reflect a combination of a decrease in popularity of the method together with the use of modern devices with longer lifespans which need refitting less often. All six devices currently marketed in the UK are available in general practice.

It is good practice to keep a variety of IUDs in stock in the practice so that the patient does not have to be sent to the pharmacist to collect her device. The choice of device is often not made until the patient is on the couch and the uterus has been sounded.

Just as with the subdermal implant, described above, specialized training in intrauterine techniques is essential. Those conducting insertions should be those in the practice who specialize in contraception. It has been shown that the variation in IUD event rates is greater between individual, experienced, family planning doctors than between the different features of the range of devices. It is likely that if such wide variation exists among such *skilled* fitters, the outcome for less experienced doctors will be less favourable. Detailed training of doctors in the skills of assessment of uterine position and degree of flexion, uterine sounding and application of instruments to the cervix minimizes discomfort and the likelihood of adverse events for the patient.

The intrauterine system (IUS)

The only such system so far available is Mirena which was launched in May 1995. It is licensed for only 3 years in the UK at present, although it is known that it is an effective contraceptive for 5 years. Luckily, although it has the same frame as an IUD, it was considered a drug by the regulatory authorities and so did not have to go through the Drug Tariff system. Despite this, Health Departments have permitted claims for insertion as an IUD. There is a highish upfront cost but this is then spread over up to 5 years when a proper cost–benefit analysis is carried out.

Caps and diaphragms

Cervical caps, vault caps, vimules and diaphragms in all sizes are prescribable on FP10. An array of practice diaphragms should be kept in stock and a scrip written for the correct size when this has been ascertained. General practice patients often prefer to see the practice nurse for fitting and checking and so training is vital. Practice caps must be autoclaved between patients to ensure that there is no transfer of sexually transmitted organisms such as HIV, human papilloma virus, Chlamydia and hepatitis B (see Chapter 3). Decontamination using chemical disinfectants is not acceptable.

Spermicides

Six varieties of spermicide (in the form of aerosol foam, jelly, cream or pessary) are prescribable on FP10 and are not subject to the Drug Tariff as they are considered to be drugs. This offers a variety of choices. The pH of spermicides varies so it is worth trying another type if the patient appears to be sensitive to one product.

Condoms

The lack of provision for male methods of contraception to be supplied from general practice is a major anomaly in the British family planning service. The historical basis for this is a debate held at the BMA's annual representatives meeting in 1975. The tone of the majority of GPs at the time is exemplified by a letter to the *British Medical Journal* of the same year which included the following sentence: 'It is surely the last straw if the Government intends to insult us by filling up our surgeries with lots of louts queuing up for the issue of condoms'. More than two decades on and with the coming of HIV infection this attitude sounds rather silly.

It seems that Devon is a particularly enlightened part of Britain; a survey there showed that one-third of practices provided condoms. There will be other areas of enlightenment too. Another book in this series, *Sexual health promotion in general practice*,[60] devotes a whole chapter to the provision of condoms in general practice. Although some pilot projects have been run successfully, there is no statutory way of funding condom provision unless in the area there is a director of public health or an HIV prevention coordinator who will give financial support. Creative ideas have been found (see section on catering for young people in Chapter 3).

Methods only available in family planning clinics

The Today sponge stopped being marketed in 1994. Some clinics supply the female condom (Femidom), which is not prescribable in general practice. It is important for the PHCT to be sufficiently aware of the advantages and disadvantages of this method so that referral to a clinic can be made if appropriate.

Methods available from the pharmacist

Pharmacists can dispense certain drugs without a prescription in the category pharmacy (P) but require a prescription for prescription-only medicines (POM). At present there are no contraceptives in the category P; there is a debate going on as to whether PC4 could be recategorized but no real progress has been made in this direction. So contraceptives sold in pharmacies belong to the general sales list (GSL) category and can equally be sold in supermarkets or garages, i.e. 'over the counter', without having to go through the pharmacist.

C-film is a spermicide that is no longer available. The recently released personal contraceptive system (Persona) is a personal hormonal monitoring kit that is sold over the pharmacy counter. It measures a woman's urinary oestrogen and luteinizing hormone and calculates in a computer chip, using data on that individual's previous menstrual cycles, the extent of the fertile period – shown by a red light. Market research shows that women regard as important the attributes of a contraceptive that enable it to be non-invasive and non-systemic.[61]

It is important that members of the PHCT are familiar with the features and benefits of methods available through outlets outside the practice.

Emergency contraception

Three-quarters of all requests for emergency contraception are made to GPs. Research in the author's practice has shown that 60% of requests take place on a Monday or Tuesday so that, as with most other emergency appointments, extra service provision needs to be made on Mondays. Flexible same-day appointments or a drop-in facility are needed. Receptionists must know the 72-hour rule for the hormonal method just as for suspected shingles. Only 4% of patients presenting for emergency contraception are fitted with IUDs, but these are useful for women who present later than 72 hours after intercourse; who have had more than one episode of intercourse, who want the IUD as on ongoing method or who have contra-indications to hormonal contraception.

Vasectomy

Access to vasectomy by way of family planning clinics and hospitals is now severely restricted and consequently many GPs have under-gone training and set up vasectomy services in their own surgeries. Although some GPs are offering vasectomy to their patients, it is not a procedure which can be claimed for under minor surgery arrange-ments. It is contrary to paragraph 38 of the Terms of Service[22] to charge a fee to an NHS patient for a vasectomy. However one can offer a private service to patients of neighbouring practices, tender for part of the health authority contract, or act as an agent for one of the charitable organizations.

Fundholding practices can charge their fund a fee for carrying out vasectomies as a provider for their own patients. This can be costed out as a 'non-core' service to include heating, lighting, staff salary, consumables and a profit margin so that the cost is comparable with other local day-case prices.

Female sterilization

Access to female sterilization always involves hospital referral. Chapter 11 covers counselling for sterilization.

11

Counselling for unwanted pregnancy and sterilization

Counselling for unwanted pregnancy

By no means all unplanned pregnancies are unwanted. A woman who finds herself unexpectedly pregnant usually experiences some distress. Her attitude to the pregnancy depends on her social and economic circumstances and the quality of the relationship with her partner. About one-fifth of women are markedly ambivalent about the situation.

Any member of the PHCT who has a conscientious objection to abortion will need to declare this and offer speedy referral to a colleague if the patient requests termination of her pregnancy (see also Chapter 12). Some women are anxious that they might receive a hostile reception. They can be put at ease by being told that they will receive support in their decision.

Many women do not require formal counselling as they are clear in their minds about how they wish to proceed. To insist on lengthy counselling for such individuals is wrong as counselling is, by definition, something freely entered into and requested by the patient. The unwanted pregnancy is a time of crisis in a woman's life that is usually resolved once a termination has taken place. The majority of women make a good subsequent adjustment. However, all women need some basic advice, apart from the necessities of fulfilling the requirements of the law. There are three options:

- continue the pregnancy and offer the baby for adoption

- continue the pregnancy and keep the baby

- undergo termination of pregnancy.

Although the first option is rarely chosen these days, except by a few teenage girls, it is important to discuss it. It is also necessary to ascertain that no pressure is being applied from any quarter. This applies particularly in the case of an under-16-year-old who should be interviewed alone if at all possible.

Some women clearly need more than the time available in a consultation to talk and think things through. Particularly when they arrive within hours of learning the pregnancy test result, a 'cooling off' period of a day or two is necessary before accepting the decision as final. It needs to be pointed out that the decision is the woman's alone and that she has to live with it, and that if she opts for abortion, she can change her mind up to the time of the operation.

Women should be given some idea of the risks involved. Morbidity is low, especially in the private sector. The risk of infertility after vaginal termination is probably less than after a normal pregnancy and delivery. Mortality for a first-trimester abortion is about one per 100 000 compared with about ten per 100 000 for maternal mortality in childbirth. The risk of abortion increases with advancing gestation of pregnancy and when the woman has had previous abortions.

All women with unwanted pregnancies need to be offered contraceptive advice for the future. In the author's view, this should be discussed before referral for those opting for abortion. Contraception is a primary care responsibility and should not be left to the gynaecology senior house officer (SHO). However, liaison may be needed in the case of a woman who opts for an IUD, as this may be inserted immediately after early termination, or an injectable contraceptive given on the day of termination. Some women are too preoccupied with their distress at the prospect of an abortion to be able to make long-term plans for contraception until after the procedure has been carried out.

Some information about local arrangements for termination should be given to the patient. This applies particularly in areas of the country where mifepristone (previously known as RU486) is being used. Currently only a few women are opting for medical abortion when given the choice, although the number is probably increasing. Most still choose a surgical procedure with general anaesthesia. Those who choose medical abortion do so because they want to verify expulsion or are concerned about the risk of trauma and the risk to future pregnancies with vacuum aspiration. Interviews conducted after the respective procedures show that the medical method is more acceptable.[62]

Counselling for sterilization

In the author's view, counselling before sterilization should not be left to surgeons. The couple should be counselled together by an experienced member of the PHCT except in the most unusual circumstances. See p. 41 for the clear distinction between counselling and information-giving. A small proportion of couples will, after counselling, decide on sterilization of the other partner. Referral for sterilization is a splendid opportunity to develop a jointly-agreed protocol with surgeons.

The advantages of sterilization are:

• a lifetime of protection against pregnancy by a single action

• very high efficacy

• no subsequent medical care needed under normal circumstances.

The disadvantages of sterilization are:

• mortality

  – female sterilization by laparoscopy ten per 100 000

  – vasectomy one per 100 000 (deaths from tetanus rarely)

• morbidity

  – wound infection

  – haematoma (about 4% of vasectomies)

• feeling of loss

• reversibility uncertain

  – best figures where an operating microscope is used and no diathermy had been performed:

    (i)   tubal patency 90% success after reversal

    (ii) pregnancy 60% success after reversal (lower figures for vasectomy carried out more than 10 years previously).

When counselling patients for sterilization, one of the first points to explore is whether the couple really rejects all reversible methods. The combined pill can be used by healthy non-smokers up to the menopause and the newest generation of intrauterine devices and the intrauterine system are more effective than even the second generation of copper-bearing devices. Some younger couples have not considered such methods sufficiently seriously.

Having ascertained that an irreversible method is really wanted, it is important to check that each partner has thought through the possible scenarios of death of the other partner and death of the children. Marital stability is difficult to assess, but all couples should also consider the possibility of marital breakdown. Special care should be taken when the man is under 35 or the woman under 30 years of age and also for those requesting sterilization within a year or so of a pregnancy (delivery, termination or miscarriage). Care with counselling helps to minimize the incidence of regret. The number of requests for reversal is now substantial. An overriding concern for the health professional should however be that a couple or an individual have a right to make a choice based on full information; the professional should not apply arbitrary rules about unsuitable candidates.

From the female point of view, she is the one who has to bear the child with the associated risks of pregnancy and she usually has fewer years of childbearing potential to lose than her partner. Women are less likely than men to feel threatened by sterilization (men may fear loss of libido and sexual prowess). It is worth checking that the woman does not have an abnormal smear, menorrhagia or a prolapse – reasons for which she might later be going to see a gynaecological specialist. All these points favour female sterilization.

The chief point against female sterilization is that it usually involves a general anaesthetic. Furthermore, if sterilization fails, 4% of subsequent pregnancies are ectopic (52% after use of diathermy). Most studies show that female sterilization does not cause menorrhagia, but those women who have been on the combined pill for a long time should be warned about the possible noticeable increase in monthly loss that they might experience.

The surgeon who operates will quote failure rates for the operation using his or her technique. The rates are about five per 1000 for both female sterilization and vasectomy. The patient must understand that after vasectomy, as well as early failures, there can be late failures due to recanalization.

Consent of the spouse is no longer considered necessary for either male or female sterilization. Medico-legal pitfalls in counselling for vasectomy are mentioned in Chapter 12.

12

Medico-legal and ethical issues

Human rights

According to the International Planned Parenthood Federation, all people (adults and children of both sexes) should have certain human rights in relation to sexual and reproductive health issues. These rights are derived in large part from documents which won international consensus at four key United Nations conferences:

- the UN World Conference on Human Rights (Vienna, 1993)

- The UN International Conference on Population and Development (Cairo, 1994)

- the UN World Summit for Social Development (Copenhagen, 1995)

- the UN Fourth World Conference for Women (Beijing, 1995).

The IPPF's charter should form an absolute benchmark against which we should assess the service we provide.[63] It is important that health professionals do not exert power and control over their patients.

1   *The right to life.* This includes avoidance of risk to a woman's life through pregnancy and to an infant's life from infanticide.

2   *The right to liberty and security of the person.* This includes the freedom to enjoy and control one's sexual and reproductive life having due regard to the rights of others; also freedom from sexual harassment and genital mutilation. This consists of having control over one's own body, using any method of contraception one chooses, and the right not to have one's body interfered with against one's will.

3   *The right to equality and to be free from all forms of discrimination.* No person should be discriminated against on the grounds of

race, colour, sex or sexual orientation, marital status, family position, age, language, religion, political or other opinion, national or social origin, disability, property status (e.g. homelessness) or birth status (e.g. illegitimacy).

4   *The right to privacy and confidentiality.*

5   *The right to freedom of thought.* Includes the right of health care professionals to conscientious objection.

6   *The right to information and education.*

7   *The right to choose whether or not to marry and to found and plan a family.* These rights come from the Universal Declaration of Human Rights and the European Convention on Human Rights.

8   *The right to decide whether or when to have children.* This includes the right of access to the widest possible range of safe, effective and acceptable methods of fertility regulation.

9   *The right to health care and health protection.*

10 *The right to the benefits of scientific progress.*

11 *The right to freedom of assembly and political participation.*

12 *The right to be free from torture and ill treatment.* This includes freedom from sexual exploitation, child prostitution, sexual abuse and rape.

Confidentiality

Codes of practice are laid down both for doctors[64] and for nurses.[35] The judgement of whether patients are capable of giving or withholding consent to treatment or disclosure must be based on an assessment of their ability to appreciate what the treatment or advice being sought may involve, and not solely on their age. Reasons for incapacity to give or withhold consent are immaturity, illness and mental incapacity.

Disclosure of information, on the basis that such disclosure is essential in the patient's best interests, should only be made after telling the patient what is going to be done, then releasing only as much information as is necessary and finally being prepared to explain and justify the decision. Disclosure of confidential information to other members of the PHCT is often essential, but medical members of the team have a duty to make sure that others in the team understand and observe confidentiality.

This shift away from the simplistic 'under-16' approach by the GMC took place in 1992, but has still not got through to all GPs. Many young people still worry that a consultation with a GP will not be confidential. Some GPs refuse contraception to young people, perhaps because they are unsure of the above ethical code or of the law on consent. Where a child consents to treatment, that child is also entitled to the same degree of confidentiality as an adult, including children in the care of a local authority and those at boarding school.

Consent

There are still some health professionals who labour under the misapprehension that a child becomes an adult as far as consent is concerned on his or her 16th birthday and that under-16s are all treated as minors. It is important to understand that the Family Law Reform Act 1969 states that the consent of a person aged 16 years or over is valid, but it does not say anything about under-16s being incapable of giving consent. The Age of Legal Capacity (Scotland) Act 1991 is the equivalent Act north of the border. In Northern Ireland the age of consent is 17 rather than 16.

Two legal principles apply to children and consent:

• consent is valid provided the child can understand advice being given or treatment proposed. This ability will vary with age and the complexity of what is being discussed

• parents' rights over their children have been described by Lord Denning as dwindling; when the child becomes a young adult the control is little more than a right to advise.

The provision of contraceptive advice and supplies to under-16s is governed in English law by the Gillick judgement. Since the ruling in the House of Lords in 1985, the circumstances in which it is legal to give contraceptive advice or treatment have been laid down clearly. The doctor should seek to persuade a girl to tell her parents or to agree to his informing her parents. Where the girl refuses both of these alternatives, the doctor is justified in proceeding without parental consent or knowledge provided that:

- the girl (although under 16 years of age) will understand his advice

- he cannot persuade her to inform her parents, or to allow him to inform her parents that she is seeking contraceptive advice

- she is very likely to begin or to continue having sexual inter- course with or without contraceptive treatment

- unless she receives contraceptive advice or treatment her phys- ical or mental health or both are likely to suffer

- her best interests require him to give her contraceptive advice, treatment or both without parental consent.

Termination of pregnancy in a girl under 16 years should be per- formed with parental consent, if the girl agrees for them to be told. However, the views of the parents are subsidiary to those of the child if they refuse consent when the child requests termination or if they demand termination when the child wants to proceed with the pregnancy. In rare cases abortion may be carried out without parental consent. In these cases it is helpful to discuss the case with a defence organization.

The Sexual Offences Act 1956 distinguishes girls aged over 13 years from those aged under 13. The penalty open to a court for unlawful sexual intercourse is much higher in the latter category. However, doctors who prescribe contraceptives to patients under 16 or 13 are not 'aiding and abetting' unlawful sexual intercourse.

There is no specific lower age limit for the prescription of con- traception or any other treatment, and doctors must exercise their own clinical judgement in each individual case, based on the child's competence to consent and her physical maturity. Where girls aged under 13 ask for contraception, the doctor should probably seek a second medical opinion and ask that colleague to make an appro- priate entry in the notes.

Sterilization of those with learning difficulties

During the last decade there have been several decisions of the courts on this subject culminating in *F v West Berkshire HA* in 1989 which went to the House of Lords. Since that case, the Official Solicitor issued a Practice Note setting out specific evidence that a judge will require, much of it social rather than medical. Even if parents or guardians are clear that sterilization of the woman is in her best interests, the case must go before a judge. Social workers and the learning disability team will need to be involved. There is no point in referring such a patient to a gynaecologist until the court has heard the case.

Vasectomy

Several claims have been successful following failure by a doctor to explain the failure rate of sterilization. A consent form that mentions failure should be signed.

It is good practice to keep a small section of each vas in a histology pot. In the event of a query a particular sample can be sent off for histological examination.

Following the operation, a patient must be warned that the vasectomy may not work, and the ejaculate must be sperm-free before the patient is advised that other precautions are no longer necessary. Claims have arisen where clear advice was not given, samples were lost or patient reports mixed up.

Compensation for an unwanted child is usually based on breach of contract. The amount of compensation in the event of successful litigation varies according to the circumstances of the case.

IUDs

A number of claims has arisen following the insertion of an IUD which at follow-up appears to have been expelled – so a second device is inserted. Later, when the patient wishes to start a family, the second device is removed but the first device stays in the uterus. If the patient is over 35, the delay of a year or more before the true cause of her 'infertility' is established may have serious consequences, including the natural decrease in fertility and the higher risk of fetal abnormality and complications of childbirth.

Perforation of the uterus during insertion of an IUD is not, in itself, negligent but a failure to recognize this complication has happened may be. Similarly, the development of infection after insertion of an IUD is not negligent, but failure to take appropriate action may be. Ectopic pregnancies can be difficult to diagnose, but the failure to recognize an increased chance in those fitted with an IUD has led to a number of claims.

The combined pill

Areas of legal difficulty pertaining to the pill have included the following:

- alleged failure to assess adequately risk factors for arterial disease

- failure to monitor the patient properly

- delayed diagnosis of cerebrovascular accident, deep venous thrombosis or pulmonary embolus

- failure to warn the patient of the effects of vomiting and taking broad-spectrum antibiotics on the pill's effectiveness.

Abortion

The relevant laws here are the Abortion Act 1967 as amended by the Human Fertilization and Embryology Act 1990. The Abortion Act does not extend to Northern Ireland where abortion is not available except in exceptional circumstances, such as to save the mother's life. The current position elsewhere is that legal termination of pregnancy may be carried out provided that two registered medical practitioners agree that:

- the pregnancy has not exceeded its 24th week and that the continuance of the pregnancy would involve risk, greater than if the pregnancy were terminated, to the physical or mental health of the pregnant woman or any existing children of her family

OR

- the termination is necessary to prevent grave permanent injury to the physical or mental health of the pregnant woman

- there is risk to the life of the pregnant woman, greater than if the pregnancy were terminated

- there is a substantial risk that if the child were born it would suffer from such physical or mental abnormalities as to be seriously handicapped.

There are no time limits when the last three grounds apply.

In determining the risk of injury to the health of the woman or her children, the woman's actual or probable future environment, for example, housing and support available in caring for the child, may be taken into account.

No person is obliged to perform or participate in an abortion to which they have a conscientious objection. However, the General Medical Council (GMC) has warned against applying undue pressure on a patient not to have a termination. If the pregnant woman is married, her husband's consent is not necessary.

In 1990, Sir Stephen Brown ruled that court approval is not needed before an abortion can be performed on a woman with learning difficulties, provided that the conditions of the 1967 Abortion Act are met.

Abortions may only take place on licensed premises. At present, in England and Wales, hospitals are the only likely places to be approved. The Secretary of State for Health, however, has the power to authorize early medical abortions in clinics or surgeries under statutory instruments. The Scottish office, however, has approved the use of mifepristone in selected family planning clinics.

Negligence

Negligence is a wrong in civil law; harm caused to a patient is hardly ever reckless and wicked enough to be a criminal matter. To pursue a medical negligence case a plaintiff (the patient) has to prove, on the balance of probability, three things about the defendant (the GP) and his or her care:

- a duty of care was owed to the plaintiff

- there was a breach of that duty

- harm occurred as a result.

The standard of care deemed necessary to show that a doctor has not been negligent is laid out in the 1957 case of *Bolam v Friern Hospital Management Committee*. Justice McNair stated that 'The test is the standard of the ordinary skilled man exercising and professing to have that special skill. A man need not possess the highest expert skill; it is well established in law that it is sufficient if he exercises the ordinary skill of an ordinary competent man exercising that particular art ... He is not guilty of negligence if he has acted in accordance with the practice accepted as proper by a responsible body of medical men skilled in that particular art'.

Personal injury claims are not uncommon in family planning when compared with other specialties. It is very important to record what counselling and which leaflet has been given or have a written policy on what is standard practice. The benefits and risks of a contraceptive method should always be explained clearly and carefully, making sure the patient understands.

A consent form is necessary for those undergoing vasectomy. Ensure adequate training is undertaken for IUD and subdermal implant insertion. Always do pregnancy tests and physical examinations on those with amenorrhoea who have pregnancy symptoms, even if they are using highly effective methods: it must be remembered that sterilization itself has a failure rate. Users of depot injections are the ones to be most careful with as they are often amenorrhoeic anyway.

Intimate examinations

The GMC has recently published guidance for doctors performing intimate examinations.[65] This is particularly relevant in family planning where breast and genital examinations are regularly performed. Every year about 20 complaints are made where the doctor is accused of professional misconduct. Such cases are particularly traumatic for the doctor concerned. A seven-point plan is aimed at avoiding such complaints.

1   Explain to the patient the need for the intimate examination.

2   Explain what the examination will involve.

3   Obtain the patient's consent.

4   Offer a chaperon or invite the patient to bring a relative or friend, wherever possible.

5   Give the patient privacy to undress and dress.

6   Keep discussion relevant and avoid unnecessary personal comments.

7   Encourage questions and discussion.

Access to medical records

Since 1 November 1991 adults can request access to their medical records compiled on or after that date. The record can only be disclosed to a second party if they have the written authorization of the patient concerned. If a patient is under 16 years old (17 in Northern Ireland) and capable of understanding a parental request for access to his or her records then he or she can prevent access. If the young person is not capable of understanding, the GP or other member of the PHCT can still deny parental access if it is felt to be in the patient's best interests. Information relating to a person other than the patient should not be disclosed unless that person has consented to the disclosure.

13

The future

I feel it is important for all of us involved in family planning to think about the future. If we have a vision of where we want to go, and then think about how we can get there, we have more chance of making progress in a purposive way. Agreed, there will be barriers and obstacles, but it is surprising how these can be overcome if one is determined to work towards a goal. This is likely to prevent or mitigate the all too common 'evolution by default'.

A nurse-led service

There are already models of a nurse-led service in operation and these are highly successful. The trend in the development of specialist nurse practitioners is likely to be extended. This means that GPs will take on a more advisory and supportive role, but they cannot expect to sit back and relax! Although nurses may provide more routine contraceptive care, GP expertise will need to be maintained for difficult cases and for the determination of the direction in which family planning services are to develop.

Before nurses can extend their role fully, however, there will need to be Health Department clarification on nurse issuing by protocol. Full implementation of prescribing powers under the Medicines Act 1968 will be needed to allow appropriately-trained nurses to prescribe contraceptives.

Generalists or specialists?

Whether GPs should be specialists or generalists is an ongoing debate within the RCGP, and its conclusion currently is that GPs should remain generalists. While having sympathy with this view, I think that practices have a responsibility to offer services of adequate quality, which match up to other services patients may choose, if not in all aspects, at least to certain minimum criteria. The antagonism of some GPs in powerful positions to the family planning movement not only jeopardizes standards of patient care but brings discredit to the bodies they stand for. Surely there is nothing wrong with family planning training being taught by specialists or GPs/nurses to a basic level and then – for those nurses and GPs with a special interest who wish to train to a higher level – further training. A primary care-led NHS surely needs both.

The RCGP set up a sexual health initiative in 1996 as part of its quality network. This is evidence of a change of heart in GP academia which is warmly welcomed.

Training issues

Training opportunities for nurses are far more limited than for doctors. This has serious implications if we are going to have a nurse-led service. Health authorities and universities must expand the numbers of places on family planning courses for nurses and GPs must allow nurses sufficient study leave. More and more training will become multidisciplinary. Ongoing training will have a higher profile with expansion of Continuing Medical Education (CME) points and reaccreditation.

Accessibility

As in all fields of medicine and public services, accessibility to family planning services will increase. Further flexibility with drop-in facilities and longer opening hours will be necessary according to locally determined needs. Yes, evenings and Saturdays I foresee! This is not just to cater for young people but for a workforce under increasing pressure too. We already have surgeries on railway stations and in shopping centres; supermarkets and DIY stores may be next!

The role of the pharmacist

The pharmacist's role is likely to be extended, with pharmacists having a still higher profile in family planning service delivery. The debate about emergency hormonal contraception being recategorized from POM to P may have become bogged down, but I think eventually the pharmaceutical companies and pharmacists will see that they cannot continue to resist this development indefinitely.

Convergence of services

As mentioned on p. 50, there has been a move to make an alliance between family planning and genitourinary medicine. The 'one-stop' clinic for an STI check and contraceptive supplies may seem a useful development but perhaps more debate needs to take place. Model services run by doubly-qualified specialists are undoubtedly successful but there may also be room for other models designed at local level.

Funding

In the 1980s we had clinic cuts, then centralization, then rationalization. Now, paradoxically, despite community trusts investing in consultants in family planning and reproductive health care, there are widespread cuts in overall budgets with arbitrary decisions being made – such as all those over 25 to be excluded from trust clinic services. This latter change has been opposed by GPs as it represents a shift from one part of primary care to another, to add to the major shifts from secondary care to primary care, all of which seem to be without associated shifts in funding.

The question of funding of local services from the same pool has often been raised, rather than the existing separation into acute sector, community sector and GP sector. This would do much to create equity and would mean that those from the different outlets would have to work together – a state of affairs to be commended.

The Department for Education and Employment

As with smoking health education, unrealistic expectations are being made on PHCTs to alter behaviour when it is far too late. Individuals need education at school at an early age.

Probably the most important advance would be a joint venture between the Department for Education and Employment and the DOH, culminating in further appropriate guidance being issued to schools, instructing them to develop sexuality education programmes extending far beyond the National Curriculum requirements. Radical new thinking in the Department for Education and Employment would be needed. One would like to see all local education authorities running health clinics and health education programmes jointly on school premises. Partnerships could be developed with those agencies best able to provide services or support.

The implications of new technologies

We have already seen massive changes with the advent of near patient testing in the form of the application of monoclonal antibody technology to pregnancy testing. Persona may be the first of many high-tech. contraceptive methods to empower women and men. With Persona the outlet is pharmacy based and not in any way under the jurisdiction of the health service. Further changes are likely with the use of mifepristone; the proportion of medical abortions is likely to become much greater. The spin-off will be pressure to carry out abortions in community premises in England and Wales, as is already happening in Scotland. This will bring abortion away from acute services and one can envisage community-based day units – which are already growing in relation to the increase in operations performed as day cases.

The team approach

This is already being facilitated by health authorities and is likely to develop further. One can predict greater integration between health visitors, school nurses and midwives, even if there is no direct contract with the practice. The domiciliary tradition of the family planning movement may well be taken forward by these members of the PHCT.

Attitudes

Let us hope we can get away from narrow-minded 'them and us' attitudes between GPs and nurses or between PHCTs and trust clinics. In the past we have tended to defend the service we happen to work in and argued why it is better than other services. We have tended to be possessive of our patients and worried that they might be 'poached' by other services. How about working together with a range of other disciplines to develop high quality services which meet the needs of local (dare I say it?) clients? In the future let us hope that between all professional and administrative staff working within spheres which impinge on family planning there can be peace, harmony, cooperation, collaboration and mutual respect.

References and further reading

References

1   Ashton JR, Marchbank A, Mawle P *et al.* (1994) Family planning, abortion and fertility services. In *Health care needs assessment*, Vol 2 (eds A Stevens and J Raftery). Radcliffe Medical Press, Oxford.

2   Foster K, Jackson B and Thomas M (1995) *General household survey, 1993.* HMSO, London.

3   McCormick A, Fleming D and Charlton J (1995) *Morbidity statistics from general practice. Fourth national study, 1991–1992.* HMSO, London.

4   Birth Control Trust (1996) *Purchasing abortion services.* BCT, London.

5   Walsh J, Lythgoe H and Peckham S (1996) *Contraceptive choices – supporting effective use of methods.* FPA, London.

6   McGuire A and Hughes D (1995) *The economics of family planning services.* FPA, London.

7   McColl AJ and Gulliford MC (1993) *Population health outcome indicators for the NHS.* Faculty of Public Health Medicine, London.

8   Family Planning Association (1996 – sections updated annually). *FPA factfile.* FPA, London.

9   Rowlands S, Dakin L, Booth M *et al.* (1994) *Contraceptive use in an English rural general practice.* Paper presented at the Third Congress of the European Society of Contraception, Dublin, 16 June 1994.

10   Bromham D (1996) Faculty of Family Planning and Reproductive Health Care. *Audit Unit News.* **1**(4): 2.

11   Carne S, Day K, Elstein M *et al.* (1990) *Handbook of contraceptive practice.* Department of Health, Scottish Home and Health Department, Welsh Office, London.

12   Family Planning Service Memorandum of Guidance (1974*a*) (Issued with HSC (IS) 32.) Department of Health and Social Security, London.

13   Family Planning Service Memorandum of Guidance (1974*b*) (Issued with WHSC (IS) 22) Welsh Office, Cardiff.

14   Family Planning Services, Health Care Circular number (74)3 (1974*c*) Scottish Home and Health Department, Edinburgh.

15   Family Planning Service Memorandum of Guidance (1975) (Issued with circular letter HSS (OS1)) Department of Health and Social Services, Northern Ireland.

16   Executive Letter EL (90) MB 115 6 June (1990). Department of Health, London.

17   West J, Hudson F, Levitas R *et al.* (1995) *Young people and clinics: providing for sexual health in Avon.* Department of Sociology, University of Bristol.

18   Aggleton P, Chalmers H, Daniel S *et al.* (1996) *Promoting young people's sexual health.* Health Education Authority, London.

19   Bailey G, Gregory A and Franks E (1996) A GP response to teenage health issues. *Audit Gen Prac.* August: 18–20.

20   Allen KM (1995) *Meeting the health needs of adolescents in general practice.* Lincolnshire Health.

21   Walling MR (1995) Teenage sexual healthcare: what guidelines? *Medical Dialogue.* **439**.

22   National Health Service, England and Wales (1992) *The National Health Service (General Medical Services) regulations 1992.* HMSO, London.

23   Wheble AM, Street P and Wheble SM (1987) Contraception: failure in practice. *Br J Fam Plan.* **13**: 40–5.

24   Burton R and Savage W (1990) Knowledge and use of postcoital contraception: a survey among health professionals in Tower Hamlets. *Br J Gen Prac.* **40**: 326–30.

25   Duncan G, Harper C, Ashwell E *et al.* (1990) Termination of pregnancy: lessons for prevention. *Br J Fam Plan.* **15**: 112–17.

26   Brook SJ and Smith C (1991) Do combined oral contraceptive users know how to take their pill correctly? *Br J Fam Plan.* **17**: 18–20.

27   Bromham DR, Cartmill RSV (1993) Knowledge and use of secondary contraception among patients requesting termination of pregnancy. *BMJ.* **306**: 556–7.

28   Houghton A (1994) Knowledge of contraception in abortion seekers compared with other pregnant and non-pregnant women. *Br J Fam Plan.* **20**: 69–72.

29   Platt MT, Batchelor L and Taylor R (1992) *Young people and sexual health – a survey of views, behaviour and needs.* Macclesfield Health Authority.

30   Institute of Population Studies (1993) *Sexual health and family planning services in general practice: report of a qualitative research survey in England and Wales.* Family Planning Association, London.

31   Chambers R and Milsom G (1997) Survey of contraceptive services and extent of staff qualifications in family planning in primary care in Staffordshire. *Br J Fam Plan.* **22**: 186–8.

32   English National Board for Nursing, Midwifery and Health Visiting (1993) *Dear colleague letter.* ENB, London.

33   Department of Health (1989) *Report of the advisory group on nurse prescribing.* DOH, London.

34   Royal College of Nursing (1996) *Issues in nursing and health*, 41. Family planning and contraception in general practice: guidance for nurses. RCN, London.

35   United Kingdom Central Council for Nursing, Midwifery and Health Visiting (1992) *Code of professional conduct.* UKCC, London.

36   British Medical Association, General Medical Services Committee, Health Education Authority, Brook Advisory Centres, Family Planning Association, Royal College of General Practitioners (1993) *Confidentiality and people under 16.* BMA, London.

37   United Kingdom Central Council for Nursing, Midwifery and Health Visiting (1996) *Guidelines for professional practice.* UKCC, London.

38   United Kingdom Central Council for Nursing, Midwifery and Health Visiting (1992) *Standards for the administration of medicines.* UKCC, London.

39   United Kingdom Central Council for Nursing, Midwifery and Health Visiting (1993) *Standards for records and record keeping.* UKCC, London.

40   United Kingdom Central Council for Nursing, Midwifery and Health Visiting (1989) *Exercising accountability.* UKCC, London.

41   Drury M and Hobden-Clarke L (1994) *The practice manager.* Radcliffe Medical Press, Oxford.

42   Robbins M (1995) *Medical receptionists and secretaries handbook.* Radcliffe Medical Press, Oxford.

43   Royal Pharmaceutical Society of Great Britain (1996) *Medicines, ethics and practice: a guide for pharmacists,* no. 17.

44   Allan D and Quinlan C (1995) *Making sense of computers in general practice.* Radcliffe Medical Press, Oxford.

45   Schering Health Care Ltd (1997) *The oral contraceptive help program* (computer disk).

46   Wise PH, Pietroni RG, Bhatt VB *et al.* (1996) Development and evaluation of a novel patient information system. *J Roy Soc Med.* **89**: 557–60.

47   Organon Laboratories (1996) *DFFP Case Studies* (computer disk).

48   Wolff New Media (1996) *Your personal net doctor (Your guide to health and medical advice on the Internet and on-line services).* Wolff New Media, New York.

49   Edwards P, Jones S and Williams S (1994) *Business and health planning for general practice.* Radcliffe Medical Press, Oxford.

50   Gilligan C and Lowe R (1994) *Marketing and general practice.* Radcliffe Medical Press, Oxford.

51   Wilson RMS, Gilligan C and Pearson DJ (1992) *Strategic marketing management: planning, implementation and control.* Butterworth Heinemann, Oxford.

52   Cunningham LF and Frontczak NT (1988) Improving patient satisfaction in healthcare clinics through the use of a focus group approach.
Health Marketing Quarterly. **5** (1/2): 89–115.

53   Clinical Guidelines Working Group (1995) *The development and implementation of clinical guidelines. Report from General Practice 26.* RCGP,
Exeter.

54   Hannaford P and Webb A (1996) Evidence-guided prescribing of combined oral contraceptives: consensus statement. *Contraception.* **54**: 125–9.

55   Stokes T (1996) Chlamydia screening before IUD insertion. *Br J Fam
Plan.* **22**: 161.

56   National Coordinating Unit for Clinical Audit in Family Planning
(1996) *Starting clinical audit in family planning services.*

57   National Health Service Executive (1996) *Promoting clinical effectiveness.* 18.

58   Evans S, formerly senior registrar in public health medicine, Bedfordshire Health Authority. Personal communication, 1996.

59   Raven A (1993) *Clinical trials: an introduction.* Radcliffe Medical Press,
Oxford (out of press).

60   Curtis H, Hoolaghan T and Jewitt C (1995) *Sexual health promotion
in general practice.* Radcliffe Medical Press, Oxford.

61   Bonnar J (ed.) (1996) *Natural contraception through personal hormone
monitoring.* Proceedings of a symposium held at the XIV FIGO World
Congress of Gynecology and Obstetrics, Montreal, Canada. September
1994. Parthenon, New York.

62   Henshaw RC, Naji SA, Russell ITR *et al.* (1993) Comparison of
medical abortion rates with surgical vacuum aspiration: women's preferences and acceptability of treatment. *BMJ.* **307**: 714–17.

63   International Planned Parenthood Federation (1996) *IPPF Charter on
sexual and reproductive rights.* IPPF, London.

64   General Medical Council (1995) *Confidentiality.* (One of four booklets
issued under the heading of *Duties of a doctor.)* GMC, London.

65   General Medical Council News Review (1997).

Further reading

Andrews G (ed.) (1997) *Women's sexual health – a book for nurses*. Baillière Tindall, London.

Belfield T (1996) *Contraceptive handbook*. Family Planning Association, London.

Department of Health/Welsh Office (1996) *Statement of fees and allowances payable to general medical practitioners in England and Wales (The Red Book)*. DOH, London.

Guillebaud J (1994) *Contraception: Your questions answered*. Churchill Livingstone, Edinburgh.

Health of the Nation (1993) *Key area handbook: HIV/AIDS and sexual health*. Department of Health, London.

Loudon N, Glasier A and Gebbie A (eds) (1995) *Handbook of family planning and reproductive health care*. Churchill Livingstone, Edinburgh.

Montford H and Skrine R (eds) (1993) *Contraceptive care: meeting individual needs*. Chapman & Hall, London.

Royal College of General Practitioners (1993) *Family planning and sexual health: a policy statement on clinical service provision*. RCGP, London.

Useful addresses

British Pregnancy Advisory Service
Austy Manor
Wootton Wawen
Solihull
West Midlands
B95 6BX
Tel: 01564 793225; Fax: 01564 794935

Brook Advisory Centres
165 Grays Inn Road
London
WC1X 8UD
Tel: 0171 713 9000; Fax: 0171 833 8182

Faculty of Family Planning and Reproductive Health Care
of the RCOG
27 Sussex Place
Regent's Park
London
NW1 4RG
Tel: 0171 723 3175; Fax: 0171 723 0575

Family Planning Association
2–12 Pentonville Road
London
N1 9FP
Tel: 0171 837 5432 (switchboard); Fax: 0171 837 3034
Helpline (Contraceptive Education Service): 0171 837 4044

Marie Stopes House
108 Whitfield Street
London
W1P 6BE
Tel: 0171 388 0662; Fax: 0171 388 3409

National Association of Nurses for Contraception and Sexual Health
19 Whitacre Road
Knowle
Solihull
West Midlands
B93 9HW
Tel: 01564 770032; Fax: 01564 770069

National Coordinating Unit for Clinical Audit in Family Planning
University of Hull
Hull
HU6 7RX
Tel: 01482 466051; Fax: 01482 466050

The National Council for Voluntary Organizations has a telephone
helplines directory which includes the addresses and telephone
numbers of many helpful voluntary organizations.
NCVO/Bedford Square Press
Regent's Wharf
8 All Saints Street
London
N1 9RL
Tel: 0171 713 6161

Royal College of General Practitioners
14 Princes Gate
Hyde Park
London
SW7 1PU
Tel: 0171 581 3232; Fax: 0171 225 3047

Royal College of Nursing Family Planning Forum
20 Cavendish Square
London
W1M 0AB
Tel: 0171 409 3333; Fax: 0171 355 1379

Appendix 1 Example of a patient questionnaire

Questionnaire TAC 1. Meeting the needs of teenagers – attenders

We would like your views on the services we provide for young people so we can make them better. Could you please, therefore, answer the questions below and return the form in the envelope provided.

NOTE: We will not be able to identify you from the details given. The sealed envelope will only be opened by the study researchers.

Thank you for your help.

Please tick the appropriate box(es).

1 I am: Male ☐   Female ☐

2 I am _____ years old.

3 I came because   – of the publicity/leaflet   ☐
                        – a friend encouraged me   ☐
                        – a relative suggested it   ☐

4 Did the publicity/leaflets tell you enough about the service being offered?   Yes ☐   No ☐   Don't know ☐

5 Was the information in the publicity/leaflets easy to understand?   Yes ☐   No ☐   Don't know ☐

6 Did the publicity/leaflet seem to cover the issues you think are important?   Yes ☐   No ☐   Don't know ☐

7   Did the publicity/leaflets make the
    service seem friendly and inviting?   Yes ☐   No ☐   Don't know ☐

8   How could we have given
    you better information?
    Please specify details in box.

9 (i) I came for   – information   ☐
       (You can tick more than one box)   – advice   ☐
                                                 – 'help'   ☐
                                                 – treatment   ☐

  (ii) I came about   – girlfriend/boyfriend problems   ☐
                                                 – family relationship problems   ☐
                                                 – HIV/AIDS or other sexually
                                                   transmitted diseases   ☐
                                                 – family planning/contraception   ☐
                                                 – alcohol/drug abuse   ☐
                                                 – smoking   ☐
                                                 – child abuse   ☐
                                                 – other – please specify details
                                                   in box

10 I was given   – spoken information   ☐
    (You can tick more than one box)   – written information   ☐
                                                 – advice   ☐
                                                 – help/treatment   ☐
                                                 – return appointment   ☐
                                                 – referred to someone else   ☐
                                                 – other – please specify details
                                                   in box

11 The information/advice/help, etc. given made
  – me feel better about my problem(s)   ☐
  – me feel worse about my problem(s)   ☐
  – no difference to how I felt   ☐

12 I came
  – alone   ☐
  – with a friend   ☐
  – with a relative   ☐

13 Did you find the staff
  – friendly and welcoming?   Yes ☐   No ☐   Don't know ☐
  – treated you as an adult?   Yes ☐   No ☐   Don't know ☐
  – respected your confidentiality? Yes ☐   No ☐   Don't know ☐

14 Were the rooms
  – comfortable?   Yes ☐   No ☐   Don't know ☐
  – private enough?   Yes ☐   No ☐   Don't know ☐

15 Were the following available
  – video entertainment that you
    liked?   Yes ☐   No ☐   Don't know ☐
  – tea/coffee/juice?   Yes ☐   No ☐   Don't know ☐
  – magazine that you liked?   Yes ☐   No ☐   Don't know ☐
  – leaflets on various topics?   Yes ☐   No ☐   Don't know ☐

16 Did you find it easy to attend
  – on that day of the week?   Yes ☐   No ☐   Don't know ☐
  – at that time of day?   Yes ☐   No ☐   Don't know ☐

17 Do you think that you will come
    again if you have a problem? Yes ☐   No ☐   Don't know ☐

18 If this service had not been
    available, would you have
  – gone to the GP about your
    problems?   Yes ☐   No ☐   Don't know ☐
  – gone to someone else?   Yes ☐   No ☐   Don't know ☐

    (Who? _____)

19 What could we do to make
    the service better for you?
    Please specify details in box

20 Any other comments?

Thank you for completing this questionnaire. Please seal in envelope provided
and post.

Appendix 2 Protocol for the administration of injectable contraceptives

There are two injectables marketed in the UK. Depo-Provera was licensed for long-term use in 1984 and in 1995 its licence was relaxed to allow its use as a first-line contraceptive. It is given in a dose of 150 mg every 12 weeks. Noristerat is licensed for short-term use only and is given in a dose of 200 mg every 8 weeks.

Counselling

Detailed counselling is essential before a patient is given her first injection. Initial assessment and prescription must be carried out by a doctor.

Possible systemic effects which should be mentioned are headache, weight gain, mood changes, acne and mastalgia. Delay in return of fertility must also be mentioned. Irregular bleeding is common initially, with amenorrhoea coming later in most subjects.

Reasons for opting for Noristerat include a preference for bleeding (cf. amenorrhoea), less chance of spotting, less risk of marked weight gain, shorter duration of action if worry about possible side-effects after first injection, and more rapid return of fertility after last injection.

Timing

Injectables are started between day 1 and 5 of the cycle with immediate contraceptive effect. Alternatively, a direct switch can be made from any pill. After termination administration can be made the day of or the day after the operation. After delivery, injectables should not be started until 6 weeks as heavy and prolonged bleeding can occur in the puerperium. Injectables do not impair lactation.

Routine checks

Before the injection is given, the patient should be asked whether she has any problems she associates with the method, date of last menstrual period (LMP) or whether she has amenorrhoea. Blood pressure should be measured at the commencement of the method and, thereafter, annually. Please see 'computer contraception records' protocol for codes to use.

Injections should only be given earlier than a week before the due date at the direction of a doctor. Injections may be given up to 7 days late without any extra precautions being advised. Patients more than 7 days overdue for their injection will need an appointment with a doctor. No more than three consecutive injections of Depo-Provera or four consecutive injections of Noristerat should be given without a doctor's appointment.

Giving an injection

Depo-Provera is an aqueous solution and should be given as 150 mg in 1 ml in a pre-filled syringe. The syringe must be shaken well and the air must be released before the injection is given. Noristerat is an oily formulation and the ampoule should be placed in warm water before attempting to draw it into a syringe – it is given as 200 mg in 1 ml.

Women find the procedure less undignified if they remain seated when exposing a buttock. The injection is given by deep intramuscular injection using a green needle into the upper outer quadrant of the buttock, taking care not to angle the direction of the needle medially. Never give these injections at any other site. The buttock should not be massaged after the injection as the release from the injection site may be accelerated.

Recall

Please set the recall on the computer and tell the patient the date. The weekly report carried out each Monday gives the names of patients due for another injection that week. The nurse contacts those due who have not booked an appointment by telephone or other means (e.g. via the health visitor). It is not appropriate to ask those who have not booked a routine appointment to do so. They should be offered an early appointment there and then or told they can come on a 'walk-in' basis to the gynae. clinic. If neither of the above arrangements is satisfactory then they can be told they will be seen at any time during surgery hours by the nurse who will liaise with the duty doctor if necessary.

Index

Abortion Act (1967) 103
abortions
  charitable organizations 51
  commissioning 4
  conscientious objection to 93, 103
  counselling 93–4
  and emergency contraception,
      knowledge of 25
  financing 2
  future 110
  legal issues 102–3
  parents' views 99–100
  and rapid pregnancy testing 22
  rate 1, 2
    outcome indicators 6–7
    pill scares 13
    trends 15–16
  service objectives 28
access to medical records 105
accessibility of family planning
      services 4, 19, 35, 108
accident and emergency (A&E)
      departments 50
accountability 39, 44
action plans 69
administration of practice 58
administrative aspects of contraception
      85
  caps and diaphragms 89–90
  condoms 90
  Drug Tariff 86
  emergency contraception 91–2
  family planning clinics 91
  female sterilization 92
  injectables 87
  intrauterine devices 88–9
  intrauterine system 89
  personally administered items
      85–6

pharmacists 91
pills 86
spermicides 90
subdermal implants 87–9
vasectomy 92
Advanced Family Planning Nursing
      Course 37
advertising see publicity and
      advertising
age factors 23
Age of Legal Capacity (Scotland) Act
      (1991) 99
All-flex arcing spring diaphragm 86
anonymity 5
appointment systems 5, 19, 58
attitudes, future 111
audit, clinical 73, 74, 77–9
autoclaves 21, 90

best practice recommendations 77
breast cancer · 12, 13, 14
breast examination 37
breast-feeding 45–6
British Medical Association (BMA) 76
British Medical Journal 60
British National Formulary 57
British Pregnancy Advisory Service 51,
      119
brochures see leaflets
Brook Advisory Centres 19, 52, 119
business planning 62

cancer 12, 13, 14
caps
  administrative aspects 89–90
  claim forms and fees 26
  method teaching by practice nurse
      42
  recall 28

replacements issued by pharmacists
    53
  trends in usage 10, 11
'career women' 11
CD-ROM 56–7
CE mark 86
cervical cancer 12, 13
cervical smears 38
C-film 91
changing facilities 21
charitable organizations 51–3
childlessness, voluntary 11
chlamydia screening 77
claim forms 17, 26–8, 31
  practice managers' role 45
clinical audit 73, 74, 77–9
clinical effectiveness 73
clinical trials 82
coitus interruptus 10–11
combined pill
  administrative aspects 86
  audit 79
  bad press 12
  evidence-based medicine 75,
    76–7
  legal issues 102–3
  trends in usage 11
commissioners 3
commissioning services 3–4
Committee for Proprietary Medicinal
    Products (CPMP) 76
Committee on Safety of Medicines
    (CSM) 12, 14, 76
communication 57, 62, 81
competence, letters of 80, 81
computers see information technology
conception rates 5–6, 7
condoms
  administrative aspects 90, 91
  provision 21
  research 76
  trends in usage 10, 11
confidentiality 5, 30, 98–9
  electronic data interchange 59
  emergency contraception card
    47–8
  practice nurses 43–4
  telephone recall 29
  young people 36

consent 99–100
  abortion 99–101, 102–3
  research 82
  sterilization 96
  vasectomy 104
consultants 49
consultations 2, 57
consumables 22
Continuing Medical Education (CME)
    108
Contraceptive Education Service
    (CES)
  emergency contraception 17–18
  helpline 40
  leaflets 21, 23–5, 57
convergence of family planning
    services 109
copper-T 380 slimline IUD 86
cost-benefit analysis 5
counselling
  injectable contraceptives 125
  by practice nurses 37, 41
  sterilization 94–6
  unwanted pregnancy 93–4
crisis management 14
crude potential fertility rate 7
culture and ethnicity 3, 23

database searches 76
dedicated clinics 20
Department of Education 110
Department of Employment 110
Department of Health (DOH) 60, 88,
    110
Depo-Provera 87, 125, 126
desk-top publishing 58
diaphragms
  administrative aspects 86, 89–90
  recall 28
  trends 9
diary function, computer systems 58
Diploma of the Faculty of Family
    Planning (DFFP) 36, 80
DRCOG 80–1
drop-in services 5
  reissuing of contraceptives 39
  run by practice nurses 20
  young people 19, 20
drug interactions 52, 57

Drug Tariff 86
Dutch caps *see* caps

ectopic pregnancies 102
education *see* health education; sex
        education; training
electronic data interchange 58–60
E-mail 60
emergency contraception
    accident and emergency
        departments 50
    administrative aspects 91–2
    audit kit 78
    card 47, 48
    guidelines 17–18
    gynaecology departments 49
    patients' knowledge of 25
    pharmacists 52
    practice nurses 41
    receptionists' role 41, 47, 92
English National Board 36, 37
equipment 21
ethical issues
    clinical trials 82
    confidentiality 98–9
    consent 99–100
    practice nurses 44
    sterilization of people with learning
        difficulties 101
ethnicity and culture 3, 23
evaluation of family planning services
        66–8
evidence-based medicine 74–7
expanding family planning services 30

Faculty of Family Planning and
        Reproductive Health Care 49,
        119
    Clinical and Scientific Committee
        76
    guidelines 17
    Letter of Competence in
        Postgraduate Education 81
    research 82
    training of GPs 80
Family Law Reform Act (1969) 99
Family Planning Association (FPA) 80,
        119
    leaflets 52

family planning clinics
    administrative aspects 91
    alternatives to pill 25
    commissioning services 4
    doctors 15
    method teaching 25
    training 17
    trends 9
    young people 20
faxes 14, 55
fee claims 26–8, 31
    pregnant patients 46
    subdermal implants 88
female condoms (Femidom) 76, 91
female GPs 5
female sterilization
    administrative aspects 92
    commissioning 4
    counselling 94–6
    disadvantages 95, 96
    gynaecologists 49
    learning difficulties, people with
        101
    protocols 18
Femidom 76, 91
fertility rate, crude potential 7
financial issues
    abortion 2
    cost-benefit analysis of family
        planning services 5
    future 109
    setting up a family planning service
        30–1
fittings, surgery 21
focus groups 67–8
FP10 39, 40
FP1001 claim form 26
FP1002 claim form 26
FP1003 claim form 26
fundholding GPs
    abortion 28
    business plan 62
    commissioning services 4
    needs assessment 3
    vasectomies 92
furniture, surgery 21
future of family planning services 107
    accessibility 108
    attitudes 111

convergence of services 109
Departments of Education and
    Employment 110
funding 109
generalists versus specialists 107–8
new technologies 110
nurse-led service 107
pharmacists 109
planning 68–70
team approach 110–11
training issues 108

General Medical Services Committee
    (GMSC) 86, 88
general practitioners
    administrative aspects of
        contraception 85
    alternatives to pill 25
    attitudes towards practice nurses 34
    average income 31
    commissioning services 4
    discussion of contraceptive
        difficulties 15
    emergency contraception, patients'
        knowledge of 25
    female 5
    future of family planning services
        107–8
    injectable contraceptives 125, 126
    method teaching 25
    needs assessment 3
    pill scares 14
    reissuing of contraceptives by
        practice nurses 39, 40
    research 82
    schools, talks 51
    teaching 81–2
    training 17, 80–1
        future 108
        intrauterine devices 89
        subdermal implants 88
    training of practice nurses 37
    trends in family planning 9, 11
    women's choice of service 18
    see also fundholding GPs; non-
        fundholding GPs
genitourinary medicine (GUM) 50,
    109
geography of practice area 3

Gillick judgement 99–100
GMS3 claim form 26
GMS4 claim form 26, 27
GP102 claim form 26
GP103 claim form 26
GP104 claim form 26
GPC claim form 26
graphical user interface systems 56
guidelines
    administration of injectables
        125–7
    practice nurses 40, 44
    quality issues 73, 74
    setting up a family planning service
        17–18
gynaecologists 49

Handbook of contraceptive practice
    17
health authorities 51
    audit 78
    contracts with charitable
        organizations 52
    market intelligence 67
health checks 19
health education 6, 11, 110
    see also sex education
Health of the Nation 5
health promotion rooms 29
health promotion units 51
health visitors 45–6
helplines 40
    Brook Advisory Centres 52
    discussion of contraceptive
        difficulties 15
    pill scares 14
    receptionists' role 47
HIV 11
home pregnancy tests 22, 52
Human Fertilization and Embryology
    Act (1990) 102

ideal family planning service 4–5
implants 29, 87–8
    see also Norplant
implementation programmes 74
improving family planning services 30
    see also planning for patient-centred
        care

information technology
  consultation 57
  electronic data interchange 58–60
  faxes 14, 55
  implementation programmes 74
  practice administration 58
  prescribing 52, 57
  recall systems 28, 29
  training 58
  trends in general practice computing
    55–7
informed consent see consent
injectable contraceptives
  administrative aspects 87
  protocols 125–7
  recall 28–9
  reissuing by practice nurses 40
Institute of Psychosexual Medicine 80
instruments 21
International Classification of Diseases
    (ICD) codes 56
Internet 59–60
intimate examinations 104–5
Intranet 59
intrauterine devices (IUDs)
  and abortion 94
  administrative aspects 86, 88–9
  bad press 12
  chlamydia screening 77
  claim forms and fees 26–8
  emergency contraception 92
  legal issues 101–2
  practice nurses 37
  recall 29
  research 76
  trends 9, 10
intrauterine system (IUS)
  administrative aspects 86, 89
  recall 29
  research 76
item of service fees 26–8, 31
item of service multiclaim forms 26,
    27, 31

Joint Committee for Postgraduate
    Training in General Practice
    (JCPTGP) 80
Joint Committee on Contraception 80,
    81

Jordan WM 75
journals 67
Just 17 52

Lancet 60
layout, surgery 21
leaflets 42, 71
  Contraceptive Education Service
    21, 57
  emergency contraception 47
  Family Planning Association 23–5,
    51, 52
  practice 29, 71
learning difficulties, people with
  abortion 103
  sterilization 102
legal issues
  abortion 102–3
  access to medical records 105
  combined pill 102
  consent 99–100
  intimate examinations 104
  intrauterine devices 101–2
  negligence 103–4
  practice nurses 44
  sterilization of people with learning
    difficulties 101
  subdermal implants 88
  vasectomy 101–2
levonorgestrel IUS (Mirena) 86, 89
Links project 58
local factors, needs assessment 3

magazines 11, 52
Marie Stopes clinics 51, 119
market research 66–8
media 11–12
Medical Devices Agency 21
Medical Devices Regulations 86
medical records, access to 105
Medicines Act (1968) 39, 52–3, 107
medico-legal issues see legal issues
MedLine 76
medroxyprogesterone acetate (Depo-
    Provera) 87, 125, 126
method teaching 23–5, 42
midwives 46
mifepristone 94, 110
Mini-Gravigard device 86

Mirena 86, 89
monitoring of patients 23
monoclonal antibody technology 110
More 52
MRCGP certificate 80
MS-DOS 55
MULTI1 claim form 26
myocardial infarction 13

National Association of Nurses for
      Contraception and Sexual
      Health 120
National Audit Office 78
National Coordinating Unit for Clinical
      Audit in Family Planning 60,
      78, 120
National Council for Voluntary
      Organizations 120
needs assessment 2–3, 5
negligence 102, 103–4
networking 67
newsletters
   market intelligence 67
   practice 29, 58, 71
NHSnet 59
NHSweb 59
non-fundholding GPs 3, 28, 62
norethisterone oenanthate (Noristerat)
      87, 125, 126
Norplant
   administrative aspects 87–8
   bad press 12
   practice nurses 37
   research 76
Northern Ireland National Board 36

objectives
   of abortion services 28
   of family planning services 68–9
Office of Population, Censuses and
      Surveys (OPCS) codes 56
opening hours 19, 35
opportunistic family planning services
      20
opportunities for family planning
      services 64, 65
oral contraception see pill
Oral Contraceptive Help Program 56
Organon 58

outcome indicators 6–8, 73, 77–8
outlets for contraceptive supplies 9–10
over-the-counter (OTC) contraceptives
      52

parental access to medical records
      105
parental consent 19, 101
patient-centred care see planning for
      patient-centred care
Patient wise 57
pelvic examination 37
performance indicators 6–8, 73,
      77–8
personal computers (PCs) 56–7
personal contraceptive system
      (Persona) 91, 110
personal injury claims 104
pharmaceutical representatives 42, 67
pharmacists 52–3, 91, 109
Pharmacy Healthcare Scheme 52
pill
   administrative aspects 86
   alternatives, provision of 25
   audit 78–9
   checks by practice nurses 39
   criticisms of general practice 85–6
   evidence-based medicine 75, 76–7
   information technology 56
   method teaching 23
   recall 28
   reissuing 39, 47
   repeat prescribing 57
   scares 11, 12–14, 76
      information technology 14, 55,
      58
   side-effects 12–14, 75
   supplied by pharmacist 53
   trends in usage 10, 11
   see also combined pill;
      progestogen-only pill
planning for patient-centred care 61–2
   current situation 62–8
   future of service 68–70
   promotion 70–1
   rewards 71
posters 29, 58, 71
   telephone advice 40
practice leaflets 29, 71

practice manager 45
practice newsletters 29, 58, 71
Practice Nurse Association 33
practice nurses
  accessibility 35
  confidentiality 43–4
  contraceptive reissues 39–40
  counselling 41
  development of practice nursing 33
  discussion of contraceptive
    difficulties 15
  drop-in services 20
  education 36–8
  emergency contraception 40–1
  female barrier methods 42
  future of family planning services
    107
  ideal family planning services 5
  legal issues and accountability 44
  pill checks 39
  as resource 42
  role development 38
  teaching 81–2
  teamwork 42–3
  telephone advice 40
  training 33, 34, 36–8
    caps and diaphragm 90
    counselling 41
    future 108
  trends in family planning
    services 9
  underused and undervalued 34
  women's choice of service 18
  young people 35–6
pregnancy testing
  home 22, 52
  monoclonal antibody therapy 110
  by pharmacists 52
  same-day 22
premises 21
prescribing 85–6
  information technology 57
  by pharmacists 52–3
  by practice nurses 39–40, 107
primary health care team (PHCT)
  computer systems 55
  confidentiality 36, 98–9
  conscientious objection to abortion
    93

discussion of contraceptive
    difficulties 16
  needs assessment 3
  pharmacists 52
  planning for the future 69
  promotion of family planning
    services 70–1
  protocols, introduction of 74
  sexually transmitted infections 50
  training 46, 81
  women's choice of service 18
privacy 5, 21, 30
processes in family planning services
    77
progestogen-only pill
  administrative aspects 86
  audit 78
  research 75
  trends in usage 11
promotion of family planning services
    70–1
protocols 39, 41, 57
psychosexual issues 37, 41
public health perspective 1
  commissioning services 3–4
  cost-benefit analysis 5
  figures for a model practice 1–2
  ideal family planning services
    4–5
  needs assessment 2–3
  outcome indicators 6–8
  targets 5–6
publicity and advertising 5, 29–30
  national campaigns 51
  practice nurse skills 34
  telephone advice 40
  young people 19, 20

qualifications
  GPs 17, 80–1
  practice managers 45
  practice nurses 33
quality issues
  audit 77–9
  clinical effectiveness 73
  evidence-based medicine 74–7
  protocols 74
  research 82
  setting standards 79–80

teaching 81–2
training 80–1
questionnaires, patient 66, 121–4

Read codes 55–6
recall 28–9, 127
  see also reissuing of contraceptives
receptionists
  emergency contraception 41, 47,
    92
  role 47
  young people 36
records, access to 105
Red Book 17, 85
registration of new patients 58
regulations 17
reissuing of contraceptives 39–40
  see also recall
religion 23
reminders 29
repeat prescribing 57
report generators 58
research 73, 75–6, 82
resources rooms 29
Review Body on Doctors' and
    Dentists' Pay 31
Royal College of General Practitioners
    (RCGP) 80, 107–8, 120
Royal College of Nursing (RCN) 33,
    40, 120
Royal College of Obstetricians and
    Gynaecologists (RCOG) 18,
    49

same-day pregnancy testing 22
school nurses 46
schools 51
Scottish National Board 36
screening 77
SES 2000 21
SES Vacuum Little Sister 3 21
setting up a family planning service
  abortion 28
  choice of method offered 22–3
  claim forms and fees 26–8
  dedicated clinics 20
  expanding and improving the
    service 30
  financial aspects 30–1

guidelines 17–18
method teaching 23–5
monitoring of patients 23
premises and equipment 21–2
publicity 29–30
recall 28–9
regulations 17
women's choice of service 18
young people 18–20
sex education 11, 51
sexual health awards 80
sexually transmitted infection (STI) 23,
  50
Sexual Offences Act (1956) 100
sexual relationship, circumstances of
  23
socio-economic factors 3, 23
software 55–7
sources of contraceptive supplies
  9–10
spermicides 90, 91
sponges 91
spreadsheets 58
standards, setting 79–80
Standing Medical Advisory Committee
  17
statistical validity of outcome
  indicators 8
sterilization
  advantages and disadvantages 95
  counselling 94–6
  family planning clinics 49
  of instruments 21
  people with learning difficulties
    101
  see also female sterilization;
    vasectomies
strengths of family planning services
  64–5
structure of family planning services
  77
subdermal implants 29, 85–6
  see also Norplant
SWOT analysis of practice 62–6

targets 5–6
teaching 81–2
teamwork 43
  emergency contraception 41

future 110–11
planning for patient-centred care
    62
training 81
technological developments 110
teenage magazines 11, 52
teenagers see under-16s; young
    people
telephone
    advice by practice nurses 40
    helplines see helplines
    recall 29
    skills, receptionists 47
temporary residents 26, 28
tenders 3
terminations of pregnancy see
    abortions
threats to family planning services 64,
    66
thromboembolism 14, 75, 76
    media reporting 12, 13
Today sponges 91
total period legal abortion rate 6–7
total purchasing 4
toys 21
tracking, computerized 29
training, family planning
    GPs 17, 80–1
        future 108
        intrauterine devices 89
        subdermal implants 88
    health authorities' role 51
    health visitors 46
    information technology 58
    practice nurses 33, 34, 36–8
        caps and diaphragms 90
        counselling 41
        future 108
    primary health care team 46, 81
    receptionists 47
travel constraints, young people 19
trends in family planning
    abortion 15–16
    contraceptive usage 10–11
    general practice computing
        55–7
    GP family planning services 9
    media 11–12
    pill scares 12–14

preferred source of outlet
    9–10
trials 82
trust providers 3

under-16s
    access to medical records 105
    conception rate 5, 7
    consent 99–100
    counselling for unwanted pregnancy
        93
    emergency contraception cards 47,
        48
    see also young people
United Kingdom Central Council for
        Nursing, Midwifery and Health
        Visitors (UKCC) 43, 44
UNIX 55
unplanned pregnancies 1, 78
unwanted pregnancies 93–4

vasectomies
    administrative aspects 92
    commissioning 45
    consent 104
    counselling 94–6
    disadvantages 95
    fees 28
    guidelines 18
    legal aspects 102
    trends 11
voluntary childlessness 11

waiting room 29, 40
weaknesses of family planning services
    64, 65
Welsh National Board 36
Windows 55
withdrawal (coitus interruptus)
    10–11
women's magazines 11
word processors 58
workstations 56
World Health Organization 60
World Medical Association
        Declaration of Helsinki 82
wrapped instruments 21

XENIX 55

young people
  centres for 50
  confidentiality 43, 98–9
  consent 99–100
  practice nurses 35–6
  questionnaires 121–4

  school nurses 46
  setting up a family planning service
    18–20
  see also under-16s
Your personal net doctor 60
youth advisory services 6